BLOOD

THE

AND IMMUNE SYSTEM

YOUR BODY YOUR HEALTH

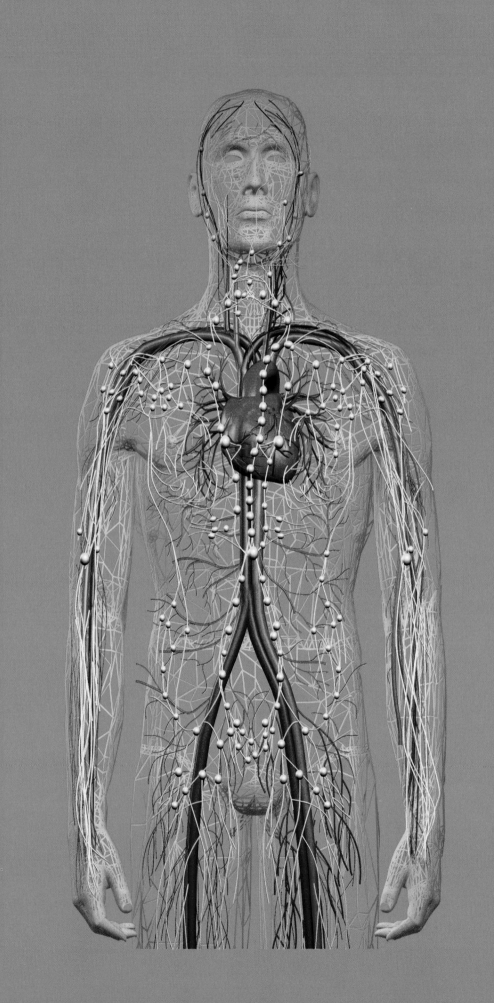

BLOOD
THE
AND IMMUNE SYSTEM

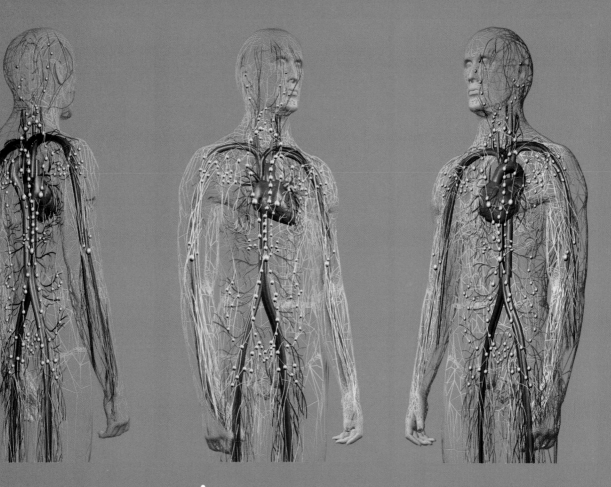

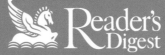
Reader's
Digest

The Reader's Digest Association, Inc.

Pleasantville, New York

London New York Sydney Montreal

The Blood and Immune System

was created and produced by
Carroll & Brown Limited
20 Lonsdale Road
London NW6 6RD

First English Edition Copyright © 2002
The Reader's Digest Association Limited
London

Copyright © 2003 The Reader's Digest
Association, Inc.

Library of Congress Cataloging-in-Publication Data
Your body your health.
Blood & the immune system / Reader's Digest.--
1st English ed.
     p. ; cm. -- (Reader's Digest home and
     health books)
Includes index.
   ISBN 0-7621-0483-X (hardbound)
1. Blood--Popular works. 2. Immune system--
Popular works.
     [DNLM: 1. Blood--Popular Works.
     2. Immune system--Popular Works. WH
     100 Y81 2003] I. Title: Blood & the
     immune system. II. Title: Blood and the
     immune system. III. Reader's Digest
     Association. IV. Series.
QP91.Y68 2003
612.1'1--dc21

                                        2003007038

Printed in the United States of America
1 3 5 7 9 8 6 4 2

IE 0004/1 C

**The information in this book is for
reference only; it is not intended as a
substitute for a doctor's diagnosis and
care. The editors urge anyone with
continuing medical problems or
symptoms to consult a doctor.**

American Edition Produced by

NOVA Graphic Services, Inc.
2370 York Road, Suite A9A
Jamison, PA 18929 USA
(215)542-3900

President
David Davenport

Editorial Director
Robin C. Bonner

Composition Manager
Steve Magnin

Art Director
Paul Fry

Associate Project Editor
Linnea Hermanson

Blood and Immune System Consultant
Dr. Alvaro Pereira-Rico, MD,
Department of Hematology and Oncology
Thomas Jefferson University, Philadelphia

CONTRIBUTORS

Dr. Wynnie Chan, BSc, PhD, Public Health Nutritionist

Chrissie Gallagher-Mundy, BA (Hons), Fitness Writer,
Director, London Academy of Personal Fitness

Katy Glynne, BSc, MRPharmS, Dip Pharmacy Practice,
Clinical Services Manager, Charing Cross Hospital, London,
Clinical Lecturer, The School of Pharmacy, University of London

Dr. Matthew Helbert

Dr. Martin L. Hibberd, PhD, Lecturer in Infectious Diseases,
Imperial College Faculty of Medicine, Department of Paediatrics, St. Mary's Hospital, London

Joel Levy, BSc, MA, Medical Writer

Mr. Gareth Page, BSc, MSc, Laboratory Manager, Clinical Transplantation Laboratory,
Guy's and St. Thomas' Hospitals NHS Trust, London
Training Coordinator for the British Society for Histocompatibility and Immunogenics (BSHI)

Jo Robinson, National Development and Training Officer,
Terrence Higgins Trust

For the Reader's Digest
Editor in Chief Neil E. Wertheimer
Managing Editor Suzanne G. Beason
Senior Designer Judith Carmel
Production Technology Manager Douglas A. Croll
Manufacturing Manager John L. Cassidy

The Blood and Immune System

Awareness of health issues and expectations of medicine are greater today than ever before. A long and healthy life has come to be looked on not so much as a matter of luck but almost as a right. However, as our knowledge of health and the causes of disease has grown, it has become increasingly clear that health is something that we can all influence, for better or worse, through choices we make in our lives. *Your Body Your Health* is designed to help you make the right choices to make the most of your health potential. Each volume in the series focuses on a different physiological system of the body, explaining what it does and how it works. There is a wealth of advice and health tips on diet, exercise, and lifestyle factors, as well as the health checks you can expect throughout life. You will find out what can go wrong and what can be done about it and learn from people's real-life experiences of diagnosis and treatment. Finally, there is a detailed A-to-Z index of the major conditions that can affect the system. The series builds into a complete user's manual for the care and maintenance of the entire body.

This volume on the blood and immune system looks at how your body protects itself. It reveals how blood is formed and the highly specialized functions of its component cell types, from iron-rich red blood cells that carry oxygen, to killer cells that conquer and neutralize invaders. You will discover the vital role of lymph fluid in guarding against infection and what goes on in the lymphatic system when an enemy is detected. The book describes what happens when people give blood and what has been done to make sure the blood donation system is safe for both donors and recipients. You will find out how to ensure that you get the nutrients your blood and immune system need, why too much exercise can be harmful, and how vaccination to promote immunity to disease has transformed health worldwide. Finally, the book discusses what can go wrong with the blood and immune system and the range of diagnostic and treatment options available today, including state-of-the-art techniques.

Contents

1

How your blood and immune system work

2

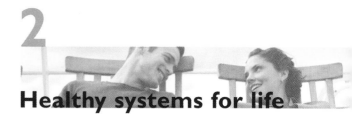

Healthy systems for life

TAKE CHARGE OF YOUR HEALTH

EATING FOR BLOOD AND IMMUNE HEALTH

EXERCISING FOR CIRCULATORY HEALTH

PROTECTING YOURSELF

3

What happens when things go wrong

The life story of blood and the immune system

The ancients believed that blood contained the life force, the supernatural energy that animated all living things. From the time of the great Greek and Roman physicians until just a few centuries ago, it was believed that there were several fundamental energies at work in the body and that blood was the medium through which these energies moved.

According to the medical system of the Roman physician Galen, followed by every doctor in Europe until the 17th century, blood delivered natural spirits (the "spark of life") and vital spirits (which provided the power of movement) to all parts of the body.

Several centuries of scientific endeavor have arrived at very similar conclusions, with the words "nutrients" and "oxygen" substituted for natural and vital spirits. Blood distributes nutrients around the body, making life possible, and, in particular, it delivers oxygen to the muscles, where it is used to provide the energy for movement. But our modern understanding, although it confirms ancient wisdom in some respects, is both more detailed and more profound. We now know that blood is part of a complex system of cells and tissues with closely linked origins and functions, a system that plays an essential role in maintaining the health and well-being of every cell in your body.

VERSATILE BLOOD

Not all living things have blood—microorganisms, plants, and even simple animals like sponges do without. But evolving a liquid medium such as blood for transporting gases and nutrients was essential if animals were to evolve any further than the level of sponges—to become large, complex, and active. Blood allows different parts of the body, sometimes separated by considerable distances—the head and tail of a blue whale may be more than 100 feet apart—to perform specialized tasks without having to worry about securing their own supplies of nutrients. Its efficiency in delivering oxygen allows animals to maintain a high activity rate, and its ability to reach every tissue makes it an essential component in the process of

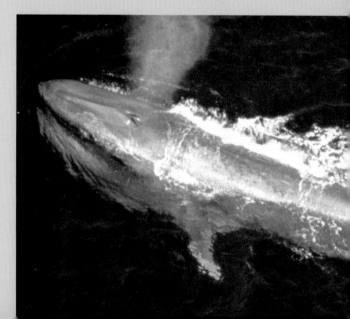

There are about 50 billion white cells in your bloodstream; their function is to protect you from infection.

homeostasis that maintains constant conditions within the body, ironing out fluctuations that could threaten to disrupt the functioning of the whole. Using a fluid medium for nutrient transportation introduces the risk of leaks, but blood has evolved its own solution to the problem of bleeding. It carries with it a sophisticated system for plugging gaps and stopping leaks.

ACTIVE DEFENSE

Your body needs more protection than simply plugging leaks in the blood supply. Thanks in part to the success of blood, your body is an attractive target for many kinds of organisms, such as bacteria, viruses, and parasites, that seek to exploit your body's resources. This can upset the delicate balance of internal conditions that your body requires. To protect against attack, you need robust and effective safeguards. Your defense system must also have other properties if it is not to do more harm than good.

For instance, a defense system that simply attacks at will would quickly destroy any cells it encounters, including friendly cells belonging to your own body (known as "self"). A defense system must therefore be selective: It must know how to tell the difference between invaders ("non-self" organisms) and friendly cells, and it must be able to target its response accordingly. To make matters even more complicated, the distinction between self and non-self is not always clear, because invaders use cunning stratagies to try to fool your defenses. Some hide inside your own cells, and others change their external appearance faster than your defenses can respond.

HEALTHY COMPETITION

Power, selectivity, and sophistication are thus the requirements for a defense system—and an effective immune system meets all of them. Competition with microorganisms has led to an evolutionary

Size does not matter
A constant supply of blood—and therefore oxygen—means that the different body parts of even the largest creatures are able to function as a whole and in cooperation with each other.

arms race. The result is an immune system equipped with an astonishingly sophisticated army of cells and proteins that stimulate, regulate, and interact with each other in ways we are only just beginning to understand. Some of these cells patrol the bloodstream, and some guard the tissues of the body. Others make their home in a system of vessels and nodes known as the lymphatic system, which filters fluids from the tissues before it returns them to the bloodstream. Your blood, your lymphatic system, and the immune system whose components they make up, are collectively referred to as the hemolymphatic system.

HOW THE BLOOD AND IMMUNE SYSTEM DEVELOP

The first blood cells appear in the primitive circulatory system of a developing embryo just three weeks after fertilization, but they are created outside the actual embryo—in a yolk sac, a developmental reminder of our shared ancestry with birds and reptiles. These blood cells derive from a type of cell in the yolk sac called an embryonic blood cell (EBC). EBCs are a type of stem cell—a cell whose destiny is not fixed but can give rise to several different lineages of daughter cells.

As soon as they appear in the embryo, the EBCs start to divide, producing more of their kind and also the first oxygen-carrying red blood cells, which make up the bulk of blood. They also produce white blood cells—immune system cells that provide the embryo with its first, rudimentary defenses against infection. About six weeks after fertilization, EBCs migrate through the primitive circulatory system to the developing liver and spleen,

IMMUNITY FOR LIFE

The immune system is fully developed from early infancy and offers protection against hostile viruses, bacteria, and parasites. Although its strength depends primarily on genetic inheritance, there are lifestyle choices you can make to help maintain its function and efficiency.

where they take up residence and set to work producing billions of red blood cells.

As new blood cells flood into the embryo's circulation, the embryo's immune system is also developing and maturing. The thymus is a lymphatic organ that helps nurture and train immune cells so that they can tell self from non-self. It first appears during the fourth week of pregnancy and slowly enlarges. White blood cells from the yolk sac, and later from the liver and spleen, migrate into the thymus and begin their training. By week 17 of pregnancy, the first fully trained and operational white blood cells emerge and begin to patrol the body, although their functions are still suppressed—up until birth, a developing baby will continue to depend primarily on its mother to protect it from invaders.

Blood accounts for about 7 percent of your body weight. On average, men have 9–11 pints of blood, and women have 7–9 pints.

The Guthrie blood test
Blood samples are taken from newborn babies by
pricking the relatively insensitive skin on the heel.
The blood sample is tested for phenylketonuria,
a rare genetic disorder.

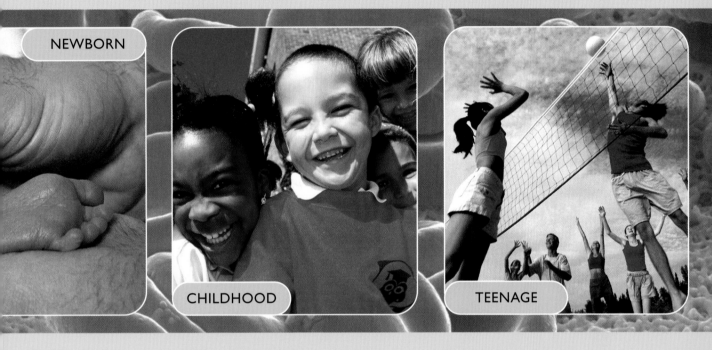

NEWBORN

CHILDHOOD

TEENAGE

Keeping disease at bay
Medical developments have allowed us to boost
our immune system's responses through
vaccination from infancy through adulthood.

Fitness first
Physical and mental health are now known to
affect the immune system, so it is sensible to
exercise regularly from an early age.

READY FOR ACTION

After about six months of gestation, EBCs in the bone
marrow—the soft, gel-like central core of each bone—
take over for those in the liver and spleen. At first, practically
every bone in the developing fetus's body is involved in
generating blood cells, a process called hematopoiesis, but
after birth, this function is concentrated in a few key
bones, including the vertebrae, ribs, and pelvis. This still
leaves the growing infant with more than enough blood-
producing capacity—under normal circumstances, a child
produces more than 10 billion new blood cells every day
(mostly to replace existing ones).

The thymus continues to grow throughout pregnancy,
until, at birth, it is much larger in relative terms than it
will ever be again. This equips the newborn to produce
lots of functional white blood cells rapidly, as its own
immune system takes over from its mother's. However,
there is a maternal parting gift in the form of antibodies—
immune system proteins that help target and destroy
threatening germs. Many proteins are too large to cross
the placental barrier between the maternal and fetal
blood, but the mother manufactures an antibody called IgG,
which is actively pumped across. Antibodies of another type,
called IgA, are passed by the mother in her breast milk
and are taken up by the infant through digestion. Despite
this lingering immune "umbrella" from its mother, a young
infant remains vulnerable for the first few weeks while its
own immune system gets up to speed, developing some
robust defenses that will provide protection and will reach
full maturity at about age five. Only in later years does the

You are what you eat
Vitamins K and B$_{12}$ are essential for your blood clotting system and the production of new blood cells, respectively.

A question of age
The immune system weakens as we age. Fewer cells are produced by the thymus gland, increasing our risk of infection when exposed to bacteria and viruses.

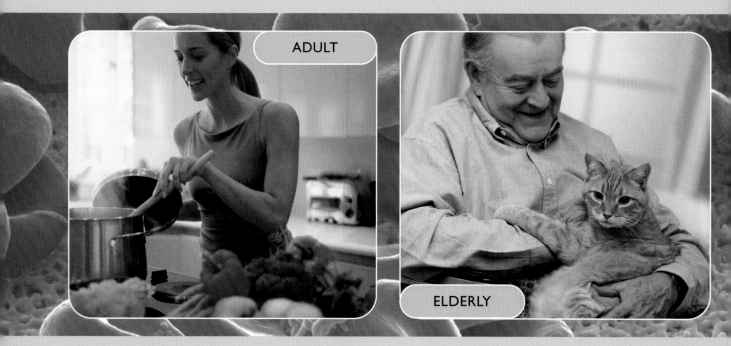

ADULT

ELDERLY

immune system begin to weaken. The thymus very slowly degenerates, fewer new immune system cells are produced to replace ones that have died, and exposure to threats produces a steadily weaker immune response. This process happens at different rates for different people—the strength of your immune system is partly determined by your genetic inheritance, but day-to-day lifestyle can be important, too.

HEMOLYMPHATIC HEALTH TIPS
Your diet affects both the readiness of your white blood cells to fight infection and the health of your red blood cells and the other blood components. You depend on essential vitamins such as B$_{12}$, found in meats and dairy products, to help you manufacture new blood cells, and your blood clotting system won't work properly if you don't eat enough vitamin K (found in cabbage, spinach, and other green leafy vegetables, as well as tomatoes and soybeans).

Exercise has been shown to boost the immune system, and doctors are increasingly coming to realize that mental health can be a powerful influence. Studies show that loneliness and boredom depress the immune system, but laughter, being surrounded by loved ones, and even the company of pets can have a direct beneficial effect on the activity of your white blood cells.

Because the blood and immune system form the basis of resistance to disease and illness of all kinds, it is important to take care of them by maintaining a healthy lifestyle—and to make full use of today's medical technology. Vaccinations such as those against polio and smallpox have given medicine some of its greatest success stories, but recent scares about the safety of some routine childhood vaccines have highlighted the need for increased awareness about issues of blood and immune health. Overwhelming medical opinion is that any risk posed by the vaccinations is far outweighed by the risks of not having them.

A person who lives to be over 70 has a 95 percent chance of needing blood or blood products at some point in his or her life.

FRIENDLY FIRE

Evidence is emerging from many different branches of medical research that the immune system itself may be responsible for some of the most serious illnesses affecting the developed world—illnesses that are increasingly common. For some of these illnesses, such as allergies and arthritis, the role of a malfunctioning immune system has been known for many years. Recent discoveries, however, have also suggested that modern plagues such as depression and atherosclerosis may be linked to an abnormal immune response. For example, according to researchers at the French national medical research agency, INSERM, signaling chemicals used by the immune system to increase immune activity are also linked to those governing mood in the brain.

Such findings suggest that the solutions to some of our biggest problems might be held by the immune system itself. It is possible that, in future, a bout of depression will be treated by an immunologist rather than a psychiatrist.

THE SHAPE OF THINGS TO COME

Stimulating the immune system through vaccination has been a huge success. Up until the 1970s, millions of people died of smallpox; this disease has now been eradicated through global vaccination. As our understanding of the hemolymphatic system advances, so does the potential for radical new treatments. Some of these are already at the testing stage: Around the world, new vaccines for AIDS and tuberculosis are raising hopes that these plagues might at last be brought under control. Synthetic blood is a long-cherished dream of the medical profession—a successful version could solve the problem of blood shortages.

The real revolutions in hemolymphatic medicine are a ways off, because scientists will not be able to manipulate and control the elements of blood and the immune system until they have a better understanding of the web of interactions among them. Once we have this understanding, new treatments for mankind's major afflictions could be produced. White blood cells could be engineered to overcome antibiotic-resistant microorganisms, the cells of transplanted organs could be engineered to be a perfect match for the recipient, allergies could be cured, and aging immune systems could be rejuvenated. This is not fiction: It is based on fact and on the extraordinary abilities of the blood and immune system.

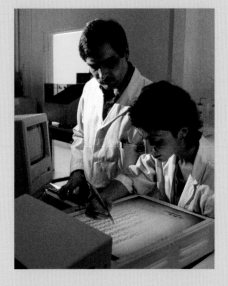

Hope for the future
Scientists around the world are trying to develop a vaccine for AIDS. HIV (below)—the virus that may lead to AIDS—attacks the body's cells' DNA. Scientists examine damaged DNA sequences (above) to advance their knowledge of how HIV and DNA interact.

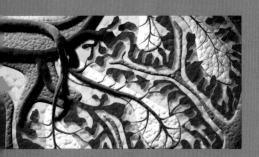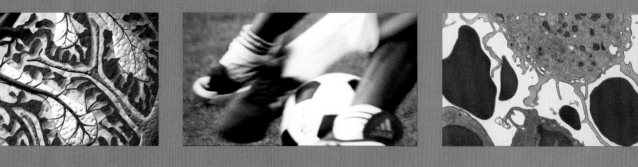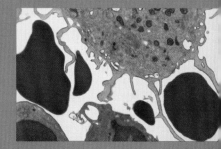

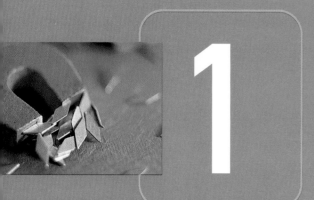

1

How your blood and immune system work

Your amazing blood and immune system

The remarkable fluid that sustains and nourishes your body also protects it from dangers from inside and out. Working in conjunction with the lymphatic system, blood provides a highly efficient defense system that fights off a multitude of invaders in order to keep you in good health.

THE FUNCTIONS OF THE BLOOD

The cells of your body require a constant supply of oxygen and nutrients, and they generate waste products that can be toxic if they build up. Oxygen, nutrients, and waste products can all move short distances on their own via the process of diffusion, but your body is too big for such a short-range process to meet the needs of your cells. You need a specialized fluid medium that can perform these essential tasks—this is the blood that flows through your circulatory system.

Functions of the blood include

- Transportation of oxygen and carbon dioxide to and from the lungs, of nutrients from the digestive system, of waste products to the kidneys and liver, and of hormones and enzymes to their target tissues.

- Defense and clotting to neutralize threats and seal off injuries.

- Regulation of pH and temperature: Your blood dilutes acid produced by working muscles and redistributes heat evenly around the body.

TO SIEVE AND PROTECT

Your blood is part of a highly evolved immune system that helps protect the body from pathogens (a pathogen is anything that threatens your body on a cellular level, such as a bacterium, virus, or poison) and filters out dead or diseased cells. Another component of the immune system is the lymphatic system, a set of vessels and structures that deals with a fluid called lymph and immune system cells called lymphocytes.

The lymphatic system *comprises vessels that transport lymph fluid and many immune cells. They follow the paths of your body's arteries and veins—see pages 28–29 for more details.*

The thymus *helps "train" cells of your immune system to tell the difference between "friendly cells" and pathogens. Pages 32–33 describe how.*

The blood circulation system *carries oxygenated blood from the heart and lungs through arteries to all the tissues of the body and then returns the deoxygenated blood to the heart and lungs via the veins. Find out more about the composition of this life-giving fluid on pages 18–19.*

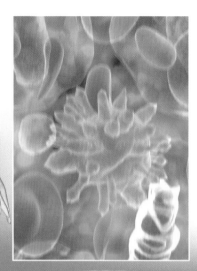

Target and destroy

Antibodies are proteins produced by cells of the immune system that are specialized to recognize and lock on to pathogens, aiding and amplifying the immune response. See pages 36–37 for more.

Small soldiers

Circulating in your bloodstream and lymphatic system is an army of immune cells known as white blood cells. The many varieties of white blood cells and their functions are described on pages 22–23 and 28–29.

The spleen is the largest lymphatic organ—it helps filter the blood and stores blood components for emergencies. Find out more on pages 34–35.

Lymph nodes—found at intervals along the lymph vessels—filter lymph and provide a base for lymphocytes. See pages 30–31.

Blood from bone

Blood is produced in bone marrow, and the pelvic bone is one of the most prolific contributors. To find out more, see pages 26–27.

Emergency repairs

If your circulatory system springs a leak, it is vital to repair it as quickly as possible. Discover how your blood repairs wounds on pages 24–25.

Workhorses

Red blood cells, also known as erythrocytes, are the workhorses of circulation, carrying oxygen to cells and picking up waste carbon dioxide in return. They give blood its characteristic color. Pages 20–21 examine red blood cells in detail.

Composition of the blood

The blood in your body may look like a liquid, but it is actually a suspension of particles in a liquid—that is, billions of cells floating in a watery fluid rich in proteins and nutrients.

The walls of an artery *are cut away here to show how they consist of a series of elastic and muscular layers. These help push blood through the artery so that blood is carried swiftly away from the heart and around the body.*

BLOOD PLASMA—THICKER THAN WATER

A straw-colored fluid called plasma makes up 55 percent of the volume of blood. Plasma is mostly water—about 92 percent of it—but it carries dissolved substances that include

- **Nutrients** that the cells of your body (including those in the bloodstream) need for survival, growth, and function. These include glucose and amino acids.
- **Waste products** that are being transported from the cells that made them to the body's filtration and disposal organs (the liver and kidneys).
- **Ions** including sodium, potassium, calcium, and magnesium. Some of these are minerals needed by cells, but in general they are there to maintain the correct concentration of blood, and to maintain the balance of other body fluids.
- **Proteins,** including albumins, which help maintain the concentration of the blood and also transport fats (which are normally insoluble in water); globulins, which have several roles, including defense and transportation of hormones; and fibrinogen, which is the inactive form of fibrin. Fibrin is a long, sticky, insoluble protein that helps coagulate the blood and form blood clots.

BLOOD CELLS

The 45 percent of blood that is not plasma is composed of a mixture of cells and cell fragments collectively known as blood cells. There are three main types: red blood cells, white blood cells, and platelets.

AN EVER-CHANGING STREAM

The mix of red blood cells, white blood cells, and platelets in the bloodstream is constantly changing as cells move in and out of tissues, old cells die, and new ones replace them. Blood loss from injury will temporarily decrease the number of cells, whereas spending time at a higher altitude will increase the number because more red blood cells are made to compensate for the lower oxygen levels. By training at high altitudes, athletes use this phenomenon to boost the oxygen-carrying power of their blood.

A white blood cell
The white blood cell in this colored transmission electron micrograph (TEM) is a plasma cell—a B lymphocyte in its mature, activated form; the cell's nucleus is shown as dark red. Plasma cells produce antibodies.

Platelets *are not really cells but rather are small packets of cytoplasm (the gel-like substance inside a cell) enclosed by a membrane. There is roughly one platelet for every 15 red blood cells.*

Plasma *is a sticky, viscous fluid because of the various nutrients, proteins, and other substances that are dissolved in it.*

Red blood cells *account for more than 99 percent of all blood cells.*

White blood cells *are much less numerous than red blood cells—there is roughly one white blood cell for every 700 red blood cells. They come in several different shapes and sizes.*

Red blood cells

As the main component of blood, red blood cells are both unusually shaped and highly specialized. They have a simple structure that is tough and durable enough to travel hundreds of miles and yet flexible enough to bend in half.

A UNIQUE PROFILE

Red blood cells—also called erythrocytes—lack the internal structures that are vital to almost every other cell in the body. A red blood cell has no mitochondria—the oxygen-burning, energy-producing structures that act as cellular generators—and no nucleus—the cellular control center that contains DNA and usually directs a cell's operations, the manufacture of proteins in particular. These structures are present when a red blood cell is born but are lost as it matures.

Instead of mitochondria and nuclei, red blood cells are packed with an oxygen-carrying protein called hemoglobin—up to a third of a red blood cell's cytoplasm is pure hemoglobin. Hemoglobin is the medium by which oxygen is transported throughout the body. Not having any mitochondria helps the red blood cell to avoid "stealing" its own cargo of oxygen, and the lack of a nucleus cuts down the cell's energy requirements because it precludes the manufacture of proteins. Red blood cells get all the energy they need from glucose in the plasma around them.

One third of the total number of cells in the human body are red blood cells. An average man has about 75 trillion red cells in his bloodstream, and an average woman has about 60 trillion red cells.

BLOOD TYPES

There are four blood types: O, A, B, and AB, any of which may be Rhesus positive or Rhesus negative (see page 58). The blood type of any individual is determined by his or her red blood cells. The reasoning behind this is as follows:

1 All the cells in your body are equipped with surface molecules that identify them as "self" or "foreign," enabling the cells of your body to recognize one another.

2 On red blood cells, these molecules are known as "agglutinins," and there are more than 50 different types.

3 The most important types are the A, B, and Rhesus agglutinins, the presence or absence of which determine your blood type. For instance, AB+ indicates someone whose red blood cells have all three of these agglutinins, and O− indicates that none of them are present.

average red blood cell lives for 120 days, during which time it travels about 300 miles on its nonstop journey through the body.

Like a magnet
The large complex proteins that make up hemoglobin are each composed of four subchains, each containing a central molecule of "hem"—an iron-containing complex that can pick up, carry, and drop oxygen molecules. It is the presence of this iron—oxygen combination that gives hemoglobin, and therefore your blood, its distinct color.

VITAL STATISTICS

- Red blood cells are disklike cells about 0.008 mm wide.
- They are 0.0026 mm thick around the edges but only 0.0008 mm thick in the middle, giving them a distinctive donut shape. This means that they can pile up on top of one another like dinner plates, to give stacks called "rouleaux," allowing many of them to pass through a vessel only fractionally wider than a single red blood cell without jamming it.
- The flattened shape of a red blood cell gives it a large surface area, increasing its capacity for gaseous exchange—delivering life-giving oxygen to the body's cells and exchanging it for their waste product: carbon dioxide. The total surface area of all the red blood cells in an average adult is estimated at about 41,000 square feet—enough to cover four tennis courts.
- Red blood cells are extremely flexible, allowing them to bend and squeeze through narrow spaces so that they can carry their load of oxygen into every nook and cranny of the body.

White blood cells

Circulating in your blood and scattered through all the tissues of your body is an army of defensive cells collectively known as white blood cells or leukocytes. Like soldiers in an army, they are trained to perform different roles and to work together to defeat the enemy.

SMALL SOLDIERS

White blood cells, or leukocytes, derive their name from their colorless appearance under a microscope when compared with red blood cells. They perform a variety of vital roles in the immune system. Some, such as neutrophils, are specialized to recognize and identify pathogens and then to relay this information to others that in turn are specialized to attack and destroy the pathogens. Some—especially neutrophils—spend most of their time circulating in the bloodstream, whereas others—such as mast cells—spend their time in the tissues of the body (known as peripheral tissues). Most move between the bloodstream and the tissues.

The type of white blood cells known as lymphocytes spend much of their time in the lymphatic system (see pages 28–29).

Monocytes
Making up 5–10 percent of circulating white blood cells, monocytes are large phagocytic cells programmed to roam through peripheral tissues looking for pathogens. They are antigen-presenting cells (APCs): When they find a pathogen, they digest it and express one of its antigens on their own surface, activating other white blood cells to hunt for that specific antigen. A pathogen such as a virus could present dozens of potential antigens, each offering a potential route of attack for the immune system.

Monocyte

Eosinophils
Making up only 2–4 percent of the circulating white blood cell population, eosinophils generally patrol peripheral tissues. They are able to attack the surface of pathogens too big to be eaten by neutrophils.

Eosinophil

Glossary

Antibody A protein molecule produced by a lymphocyte in response to the presence of a particular antigen; it attacks the antigen and renders it harmless.

Antigen A molecule—of poison, for example, or of a bacterial cell wall—that provokes an immune response. A pathogen such as a virus can present dozens of potential antigens.

Erythrocyte A red blood cell.

Leukocyte A white blood cell.

Lymphocyte A type of white blood cell that is mostly found in the lymphatic system.

Pathogen Anything that threatens the body on a cellular level, such as a bacterium, virus, molecule of poison, or cancerous cell.

Phagocyte A cell that consumes and breaks down other cells or pathogens.

Neutrophils

The most common type of white blood cell found in the bloodstream, neutrophils are short-lived, surviving for only 12 hours. They are highly mobile, aggressive phagocytes that consume other cells or pathogens. They are the first white blood cells to appear at the site of an injury, where they consume germs that may have gotten into the wound and then themselves break down and release chemicals that attract other immune cells.

Neutrophil

Mast cell

Mast cells

Permanently anchored in peripheral tissue, mast cells are filled with granules of histamine. They are largely responsible for allergic response.

Basophils

Usually found in peripheral tissues, these are filled with granules of histamine, a substance that triggers inflammation and is involved in the allergic response. They release their granules when they encounter damaged tissue.

Platelets and clotting

With 7 to 11 pints of blood pumping through your system at high pressure, the danger posed by a leak of any kind is considerable. Platelets and proteins called clotting factors provide your blood with a system of "leak control."

HOW A BLOOD CLOT FORMS

When a blood vessel wall becomes damaged and a tear develops, millions of platelets come together to form a platelet plug, which is enmeshed in a skeleton of fibrin fibers and attached to the sides of the tear. This process is triggered when a tear in a blood vessel wall exposes the collagen fibers inside it. Receptors on the surface of passing platelets bind to the exposed collagen fibers. The platelets become more crinkly to increase their surface area and stickiness. At the same time, they release signaling chemicals that attract other platelets and trigger substances called clotting factors.

The clotting factors activate each other in a series, culminating in the production of fibrin. Platelets and strands of fibrin combine into a clump that plugs the gap in the blood vessel wall. The platelets in the plug contain protein filaments like those found in muscles. After a platelet plug has formed, these filaments contract, shrinking the plug and pulling the sides of tear closer together. Immune system cells move in under the clot to clear away invading pathogens.

There are about 2 trillion platelets in the blood plus another trillion in reserve in the spleen. A platelet lives for 10 days, so every day you lose and replace more than 200 billion.

Platelets *hurry to the scene of the damage. In their inactivated state in the bloodstream, platelets are shaped like flattened disks. On activation (that is, when forming a clot) they change shape to become crinkly. This increases their adhesive qualities and also the surface area available for making contact with and binding to other platelets.*

CLOTTING FACTORS

- Clotting factors are the substances that activate and control the conversion of soluble fibrinogen in the blood into insoluble fibrin, molecules of which stick together to produce a fibrous framework for clot formation.
- There are 14 clotting factors, or coagulation proteins, that interact in a specific sequence to generate thrombin, the enzyme that converts fibrinogen into fibrin.
- Each factor activates the next factor in sequence. This series of steps helps produce a "cascade" effect, so that one molecule of factor IX (one of the sequence starting points) can eventually generate up to 200 million molecules of fibrin. The step sequence is also a safeguard against the potential danger of the clotting process forming unwanted clots that can cause strokes and heart attacks.

As red blood cells *cascade from a tear in the blood vessel wall, exposed collagen fibers in the wall attract passing platelets, which triggers the clotting process.*

Fibrin *is a strong, filament-like molecule that forms the framework of a clot, meshing platelets and red blood cells. Fibrin is held in the blood as soluble fibrinogen until required. Clotting factors stimulate its conversion into insoluble fibrin.*

The blood vessel wall *includes a thick layer of a fibrous protein called collagen. If the vessel wall is torn, the collagen fibers attract passing platelets.*

Platelets *are tiny membrane-enclosed packets of cytoplasm no more than 0.003 mm wide. They bind with strands of fibrin to form a clot. Once the clot has formed, protein filaments in the platelets contract to pull the sides of the tear together.*

Bone marrow—where blood comes from

Blood cells have a higher rate of turnover than practically any other tissue in the body, which makes the job of generating new blood cells a big one.

Red marrow bones
The bones involved in blood production on an everyday basis are highlighted here in pink— mainly the sternum, ribs, vertebrae, and pelvis.

BLOOD FACTORY

Each bone in your body has a spongy central core filled with a soft, pulpy tissue known as bone marrow, but only a few bones—primarily the vertebrae, sternum, ribs, and pelvis—contain red marrow, which produces blood cells. In red marrow, a network of blood vessels supplies nutrients to and picks up new cells from clusters of blood-producing cells called hematopoietic stem cells. Your bones contain 1¾–3½ pints of red marrow.

Red marrow is about half fat, whereas yellow marrow, found in most other bones, is almost all fat. Yellow marrow, however, does contain a small number of dormant hematopoietic cells, which can be reactivated if your body needs to generate large amounts of new blood cells—after blood loss from an injury, for example.

Blood cell production is controlled by hormones. A hormone called erythropoietin (EPO)—recently in the news because of its abuse by athletes—can convert yellow marrow into red and increase the rate of red blood cell production tenfold.

BLOOD LINE

Hematopoietic stem cells are cells that, unlike most of the ones in your body, have not differentiated into particular cell types and have the capacity to produce many different cell types. The most common hematopoietic cells are erythroblasts, which produce red blood cells. Other types give rise to different classes of white blood cell or to platelet-producing cells.

Vein

An osteon
—also known as a haversian system— is one of the cylindrical units of which compact bone is made. At the center of each osteon is a canal along which run blood vessels and nerves.

Red marrow produces about 3 million new red blood cells every second. Under stimulation by the hormone erythropoietin, this can increase to an amazing 30 million per second.

Bone

Bone is the hard, dense, connective tissue that forms the skeleton of the body. It is chiefly composed of collagen fibers, which confer resilience, and bone salts (chiefly calcium carbonate and calcium phosphate), which give the bones their rigidity. Bone marrow is contained in the central canal.

The blood vessels *that snake through marrow are known as sinusoids. Red blood cells and platelets pass through gaps in the sinusoid lining.*

Bone marrow *is found in the medullary cavity, also known as the central canal, that runs down the center of a bone. The cavity also contains spongy bone, blood vessels, and nerves.*

**Medullary cavity
(central canal)**

Artery

The blood-producing cells *in the bone marrow gather in clusters known as hematopoietic clusters. These are supported by a framework of tissues made from fibroplastic cells that run through the bone marrow.*

Spongy bone *within the medullary canal consists of a network of narrow bars of bony tissue called trabeculae. The interconnecting spaces within the trabeculae are filled with marrow.*

Compact or cortical bone *—which lies between the periosteum and the medullary cavity—consists of many densely packed osteons.*

The periosteum *is the layer of dense connective tissue that covers the surface of a bone.*

BLOOD-PRODUCING CELLS

Hematopoietic stem cells may be divided into several different types.
- Erythroblasts: red-cell stem cells, which produce red cells.
- Myeloblasts: granulated cell stem cells, which give rise to white blood cells that can be subdivided into neutrophils, eosinophils, and basophils.
- Lymphoblasts: lymphocyte stem cells that give rise to lymphocytes. Lymphoblasts migrate to lymphoid organs such as the spleen and thymus, where lymphocytes are produced and mature.

In addition, there are large cells in the bone marrow called megakaryocytes that produce platelets. A megakaryocyte produces a platelet by pinching off part of itself.

A macrophage at work
There is a macrophage at the center of each hematopoietic cluster in the bone marrow. Macrophages help clear away the debris of cell formation, such as nuclei lost from red blood cells as they mature. They also store iron, which they transfer to red blood cells. This colored transmission electron micrograph (TEM) shows a macrophage engulfing a red blood cell.

The lymphatic system

Blood is not the only fluid circulating around your body. Complementing the circulatory system and running parallel to much of it is a system of vessels and organs that transports lymph fluid and provides a home to many immune cells.

The right lymphatic duct *collects lymph from the right side of the body above the diaphragm and empties it into the right subclavian vein.*

Thymus

The thoracic duct *collects lymph from parts of the body below the diaphragm and from the left side of the body above the diaphragm. This lymph drains into the left subclavian vein.*

Lymphatic organs *include the spleen, the thymus, and the numerous lymph nodes. They house and train immune cells, such as B and T lymphocytes.*

Lymph nodes *are strung in series along the more central lymph vessels. These nodes help filter and clean the lymph before it passes back into the bloodstream.*

The spleen *is the largest of the lymphatic organs.*

Lacteals *are large lymph vessels in the intestines that collect and transport fats.*

Lymphatic vessels *can be distinguished from blood vessels by their color. Arteries are usually bright red, veins are dark red, and lymphatic vessels are pale gold in color.*

Tiny blind-ended lymphatic capillaries *stretch into every part of the body's peripheral tissues to allow the drainage of lymph fluid. These merge into larger lymph vessels that pass through numerous lymph nodes to clean the fluid prior to its reentry into the blood.*

Up to 14 pints of lymph flow through your lymphatic system every day.

FLUID ASSETS

Tiny blood vessels called capillaries deliver blood to the peripheral tissues. As the capillaries narrow, the blood pressure inside them increases, squeezing plasma through pores in the capillaries into the surrounding tissue. This fluid now becomes interstitial fluid. Most interstitial fluid rejoins the bloodstream by leaking back into the capillaries that drain the peripheral tissues. The rest drains off by another route—the system of lymphatic vessels. This fluid is now called lymph and is similar to blood plasma but generally has a lower concentration of proteins.

DRAINAGE SYSTEM

Your lymphatic system has two main functions. One is to nurture, train, and maintain a population of immune cells. These are lymphocytes (types of white blood cells) that provide specific immunity—the main line of defense against bacterial and viral infections and tumors. They spend much of the time in the lymphatic system but cross into the bloodstream as required.

The other purpose is to return lymph to the bloodstream so that blood volume is maintained. This is achieved via a system of vessels, which starts with blind-ended lymphatic capillaries in the peripheral tissues. These merge to form larger vessels, which empty into two main lymphatic collecting ducts in the trunk of the body. The ducts return lymph to the bloodstream by draining into the subclavian veins. Unlike the vessels that transport blood, your lymphatic system is not a circulatory system—it is a drainage system.

One-way traffic
Your blood circulation is powered by the heart and by the elastic, muscular artery walls. Your lymphatic system has neither of these. Pressure from the buildup of interstitial fluid and energy from muscle movements provide the driving force, and a system of valves keeps lymph flowing in the right direction.

Interstitial fluid *enters the lymph vessel from surrounding tissue. Once inside the vessel, the liquid is known as lymph.*

An open valve *allows lymph fluid to pass through.*

Direction of flow *of lymph fluid.*

Cross section of a lymph vessel

A closed valve *prevents lymph fluid from flowing back the way it came.*

LYMPHOCYTES

- **Natural killer (NK) cells** *are lymphocytes that patrol for cancerous or virus-infected cells. When they find one they blast it with corrosive enzymes.*
- **B lymphocytes (B cells)** *turn into plasma cells—antibody producing factories—when activated. Each B cell is specialized to produce a specific antibody.*
- **T lymphocytes (T cells)** *come in three varieties:*
  Cytotoxic T cells (CTL) *attack and kill pathogens that have been identified by the immune system—for example, ones tagged by antibodies—in the same way as NK cells.*
  Helper T cells (TH) *stimulate B lymphocytes to mature into plasma cells.*
  Suppressor T cells (TS) *suppress B-cell activity, helping to prevent immune responses from getting out of hand.*

TWO-PRONGED ATTACK

The army of white blood cells in your body provides you with two types of immune response.
- **Innate immunity** *Cells such as neutrophils and NK cells patrol the body looking for pathogens. They don't need to be specifically primed—they will attack any suspicious antigens.*
- **Specific immunity** *T and B lymphocytes, together with antibodies, provide specific immunity. This type of immune response recognizes and responds to specific antigens and is able to give a bigger, faster, and more effective response. It is also known as adaptive immunity, because B lymphocytes remember antigens they have encountered in the past and trigger an even bigger and more efficient immune response if the antigens ever reappear.*

Lymph nodes

If your body is a fortress and your immune system is an army guarding its walls, then lymph nodes are the barracks and watchtowers where that army makes its home and keeps watch for enemies—germs, cancerous cells, and toxins—that threaten your health.

TOUR OF DUTY

After production and training in the bone marrow or thymus, lymphocytes enter the circulation to begin the fight against invaders and potential threats to health. They circulate within lymph fluid and in the bloodstream, and from here they cross over to one of several possible destinations composed of lymphoid tissue:

- The lymph nodes—small swellings found at intervals along the lymph vessels.
- Mucosa-associated lymphoid tissues (MALTs) such as the tonsils or the spleen, collectively called the peripheral lymphoid organs.

Lymphocytes take up temporary residence in these places and continually return to the bloodstream to recirculate and begin another tour of duty elsewhere.

READY FOR ACTION

Lymph nodes and MALTs act as checkpoints and barracks: They filter lymph before it gets back into the bloodstream and provide a base for a constantly but slowly changing population of lymphocytes. All types of lymphocytes live inside a node and are exposed to lymph as it drains through the passages of the node. If their specific target antigen comes through the lymph node, lymphocytes are activated and start to proliferate, signaling the start of the specific immune response.

Lymph nodes can be up to 1 in. wide. There are more than 100 in your body.

A tough capsule *surrounds the node.*

Section through a lymph node
The network of connective tissue that holds the lymph node together—made up of reticulin fibers—shows up as yellow in this colored scanning electron micrograph (SEM). Among the fibers are white blood cells (seen here as green and yellow spheres) in various stages of development.

Inside a lymph node

Lymph nodes are small, oval organs distributed around the body, often in a chain following a lymph vessel. They vary in size from .04–1 in. but all have a similar structure, comprising three main layers inside a tough outer capsule:

- An outer cortex where lymph flows in and which houses mainly B cells. These are organized into primary follicles, which wait for antigens to flow past. When one does, the B cells are activated and form secondary follicles, proliferating and generating antibodies.
- A paracortex that contains antigen-presenting cells (APCs) and T cells. Phagocytes that also act as APCs line the channels through the lymph node.
- A medulla containing a mixture of B and T cells and phagocytes.

Lymph percolates through these layers and then out through an efferent lymphatic vessel.

Afferent lymph vessel

Interstitial fluid *enters the lymph vessel from surrounding tissue.*

Direction of flow *of lymph fluid.*

An afferent lymph vessel *along which lymph fluid enters the node.*

Afferent lymph vessel

The medulla *at the center of the node contains a mixture of B cells and T cells.*

How lymph fluid travels through a lymph node
Several afferent lymph vessels bring lymph to the node and feed through the capsule into the outer cortex. Lymph then percolates through the various layers of the node toward the efferent lymph vessel.

Trabeculae *form the meshwork of fibrous partitions that provide the framework for the node.*

B cells in the outer cortex

T cells within the paracortex
The paracortex also contains antigen-presenting cells (APCs).

Artery

Vein

An efferent lymph vessel *carries lymph fluid away from the node.*

31

The thymus

T lymphocytes are highly specialized immune cells trained to attack specific antigens, but how do they get that way? An organ called the thymus takes raw, unschooled lymphocytes and turns them into lean, mean fighting machines.

CENTER STAGE

The thymus is relatively larger in a baby than in an adult because it must work hard to provide the vulnerable child with a population of working lymphocytes. At puberty it reaches its full weight, about ¾ ounce. From birth until puberty, the thymus is deep red in color because of its rich blood supply, but it becomes increasingly yellow with age as lymphoid tissue is gradually replaced with fibrous and fatty tissue. The degeneration of the thymus may be linked to a gradual decline in immune capability.

SUBJECT SELECTION

Before lymphocytes can provide specific immunity, they have to be trained to recognize specific antigens and to distinguish between foreign antigens (non-self) and ones on the surface of the body's own cells (self). B lymphocytes (also called B cells) are trained in the bone marrow before being released into the bloodstream (although the "B" refers not to the bone but to an organ in birds, called the bursa of Fabricus, where these cells were first identified). T lymphocytes (also called T cells), although initially produced in the bone marrow, are trained in the thymus.

The thymus is a gland made of two oval-shaped lobes situated in the center of the chest, usually just behind the sternum but in front of the heart and the major blood vessels. The two lobes are joined by connective tissue.

Each lobe of the thymus is divided into .08-in.-wide lobules by fibrous partitions called septae.

A fibrous capsule covers the thymus and separates it into two lobes. Each lobe of the thymus has an outer cortex and an inner medulla.

The capillaries that supply blood to the thymus have unusually nonporous walls to prevent antigens in the bloodstream from getting to the immature T cells and triggering them before they are fully trained. This is known as the blood–thymus barrier.

Left lung

Left lobe

Right lobe of the thymus

Heart

Diaphragm

Vena cava

Aorta

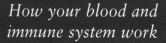
Survival of the fittest—training camp for T cells

Immature lymphocytes travel from the bone marrow to the thymus via the bloodstream. As they journey through the thymus, they face a rigorous process that transforms the fittest into T lymphocytes.

1 *Immature T lymphocytes from the bone marrow enter the bloodstream to embark on their journey to the thymus.*

2 *The immature T lymphocytes enter a lobule of the thymus via the cortex, at which point they become known as thymocytes. As soon as they enter the cortex, thymocytes start to divide rapidly, but only 5 percent make it through to the other side of the cortex. The rest (including those that might attack the body's own cells) are weeded out by nurse cells that live in the cortex.*

3 *As the surviving thymocytes move through the thymus, they are exposed to a cocktail of hormones and growth factors, including thymosin-α, thymulin, and thymopoietin. These help them mature into antigen-specific cells—cells that can recognize and respond to a specific antigen—that are ready to take up their vital role in the immune system. The mature T lymphocytes eventually enter the medulla and migrate through the walls of tiny blood and lymph vessels to other areas of the circulatory system, where they await the call for action.*

The spleen

In addition to the millions of blood cells that die or are damaged every day, the blood picks up pathogens from the skin, intestines, lungs, and many other places. The job of filtering out all this waste material falls to the spleen.

BAG OF BLOOD

The spleen is the largest lymphoid organ in the body. It is supplied with a great many blood vessels, and its high blood content gives it a deep red color. Unfortunately, the spleen is quite vulnerable and easily ruptured. Lying along the side of the stomach between the stomach, ribs, and diaphragm, the spleen is not well protected against injury. In addition, it is encased in only a thin capsule—a fibrous outer wrapping—and if this is pierced, it is hard for a surgeon to repair it because the spleen bleeds so heavily. A ruptured spleen may have to be removed entirely. Luckily, the functions of the spleen can be carried on by other lymphoid tissues, although a person without a spleen is far more likely to catch infections.

PULP FACTS

The spleen performs a function for the blood similar to the one lymph nodes perform for the lymph. It filters out germs, dirt, and dead or damaged blood cells and functions as a base for launching specific immune responses to infections affecting the blood. Blood flows in via the splenic artery and passes through areas of lymphoid tissue called white pulp, where lymphocytes keep watch for bloodborne antigens. Then the blood flows through areas of red pulp, where white blood cells of all types clean and filter the blood. The spleen also stores millions of red blood cells and platelets as a reservoir for when stocks run low.

Stomach

Spleen

MALTS AND GALT

Along the digestive, respiratory, and urogenital tracts, lymph cells aggregate into patches of lymphoid tissue that are larger than lymph nodes. These lymphoid tissues are strategically located wherever tracts communicate with the external environment, providing a possible route for pathogens to get into the body. Mucosa-associated lymphoid tissues (MALTs) include the five tonsils on the wall of the pharynx as well as the spleen. They also include gut-associated lymphoid tissue (GALT), found along the intestines, which secretes antibodies into the intestine to help fight off bacteria that try to enter the bloodstream by crossing the intestinal walls.

The spleen can store up to 5 million red blood cells.

White pulp *is lymphoid tissue. As blood passes through areas of white pulp in the spleen, lymphocytes in the white pulp keep watch for bloodborne antigens that may trigger the immune system to deal with an infection. About a quarter of the body's entire store of lymphoid tissue is in the spleen.*

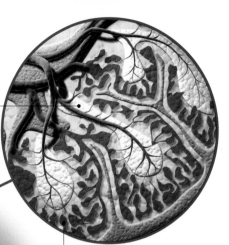

Red pulp *makes up three quarters of the spleen. It derives its color from the high concentration of red blood cells it contains, but it is white cells in the red pulp that have the task of cleaning and filtering the blood.*

The splenic artery *is the principal highway through which blood travels into the spleen.*

The splenic vein *drains blood away from the spleen and into the venous system that carries it towards the heart.*

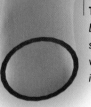

The largest lymphoid organ in the body
About 5 in. long, the spleen normally weighs about 5 oz, although in its capacity as a blood reserve it can hold as much as two pints, and therefore weigh over 2.2 lb.

Antibodies

If white blood cells are like soldiers, antibodies are the weapons they use—weapons of simple design but incredible sophistication, individually tailored to hunt, target, and destroy anything that threatens your health.

FORM AND FUNCTION

Antibodies, technically called immunoglobulins (shortened to Ig), are large proteins produced by mature B lymphocytes (often called B cells). They help the immune system recognize and target antigens and also help directly in the attack. Humans have five different types of antibodies, known as IgA, IgD, IgE, IgG, and IgM, each found in different parts of the body. They have slightly different, though often overlapping, functions, but the basic structure of each antibody is very similar.

SPECIFIC BY DESIGN

Your body makes antibodies against millions of different antigens, including many that it has never before encountered, and yet each one is specific for its target antigen. Where does this diversity come from? Although each antibody has the same basic structure, key regions of each have variable structures. The genes that code for these variable regions can be shuffled and rearranged differently in each antibody-producing B cell to give millions of possible combinations—enough to account for almost any possible antigen that you will encounter during your lifetime.

LINES OF ATTACK

As soon as an antibody encounters and binds to its antigen, it can start to attack it in several different ways.

- **Agglutination** Antibodies have two binding sites (some classes have more) and so can bind to two antigens at once. With enough antibodies, groups of antigens can be stuck together in clumps, preventing them from attacking the body and making them easy targets for other weapons in the immune system.
- **Enhancing recognition** Cells of the immune system have difficulty recognizing antigens until they have formed antigen/antibody complexes, which trigger them into action.
- **Neutralization** By covering the active parts of a molecule of toxin, antibodies can render it harmless.
- **Activation of complement** The complement system is a chain of reactions between bloodborne proteins called complement factors, which leads to the production of potent corrosive enzymes that lock on to and destroy antigens.

Your body has the capacity to produce more than 100 million different antibodies.

A plasma cell—a mature B lymphocyte—producing antibodies. Each plasma cell can produce 2,000 antibody molecules per second.

MEMORIES

The immune system can remember antigens that it has faced in the past, making it more prepared to meet the next attack. The population of B cells in the blood is always changing, with new strains replacing old ones. B cells that have been activated, however, are preserved and kept on standby and are even refined so they produce antibodies that bind more easily and tightly to antigens. As a result, if you encounter the same antigen again, your immune system is able to mount a quicker and more powerful response than it did the first time.

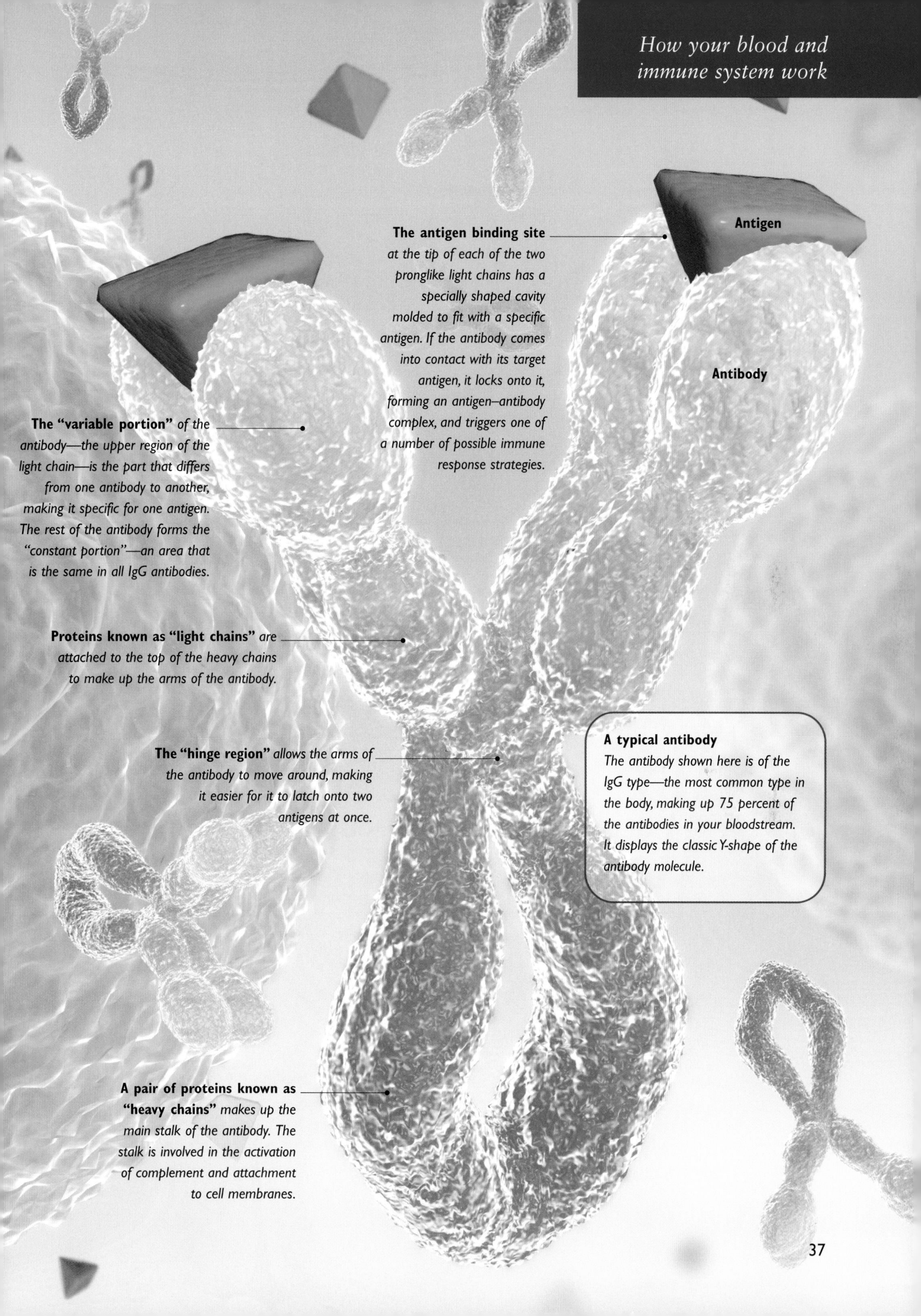

Antigen

Antibody

The antigen binding site *at the tip of each of the two pronglike light chains has a specially shaped cavity molded to fit with a specific antigen. If the antibody comes into contact with its target antigen, it locks onto it, forming an antigen–antibody complex, and triggers one of a number of possible immune response strategies.*

The "variable portion" *of the antibody—the upper region of the light chain—is the part that differs from one antibody to another, making it specific for one antigen. The rest of the antibody forms the "constant portion"—an area that is the same in all IgG antibodies.*

Proteins known as "light chains" *are attached to the top of the heavy chains to make up the arms of the antibody.*

The "hinge region" *allows the arms of the antibody to move around, making it easier for it to latch onto two antigens at once.*

A typical antibody
The antibody shown here is of the IgG type—the most common type in the body, making up 75 percent of the antibodies in your bloodstream. It displays the classic Y-shape of the antibody molecule.

A pair of proteins known as "heavy chains" *makes up the main stalk of the antibody. The stalk is involved in the activation of complement and attachment to cell membranes.*

37

A day in the life of the blood and immune system

The components of your blood and immune system interact in a complex web, as white and red blood cells and plasma proteins move back and forth between the bloodstream and the tissues, warding off potential threats from the environment that bombard your system.

ETERNAL VIGILANCE

A system as complex as your body is inevitably vulnerable to upset, and disruption to any one factor can affect others. It is vital, therefore, that your immune system is vigilant at all times, and its responses are coordinated for maximum efficiency. With such powerful biological agents, however, there's always a risk that they could accidentally attack or damage parts of your own system in an autoimmune reaction. Your immune system has built-in safeguards to prevent this, but allergic reactions are examples of what happens when these safeguards aren't working properly.

8:00 A.M. Cuts like a knife

While fixing a packed lunch, your hand slips and you cut yourself. The wound bleeds freely until you apply a bandage. Your body's leak prevention system springs into action as soon as the knife goes in. Platelets and clotting factors are immediately activated, and within a minute or so, a clot of fibrin molecules and platelets blocks the tear in the blood vessel wall. White blood cells, attracted by chemical signals given off by the clotting agents, move in around the clot and clear away any germs or dirt.

1:00 P.M. Restocking

Your spinach and ricotta salad is packed with iron, which is good because your body has been tapping its stores to help replace the lost blood cells (and their precious cargo of hemoglobin). Soon after you cut yourself, sensory cells in your kidneys detected that the oxygen carrying capacity of your blood was down and stimulated your bone marrow to churn out red blood cells at a faster rate. Meanwhile, your liver increases its production of plasma proteins. The lost blood is quickly replaced.

4:00 P.M. Summer in the city

By mid-afternoon, the pollen count is high and your hay fever starts to kick in. Antibodies of the IgE class (in the lining of your nasal passages) bind to antigens on the surfaces of the pollen grains. This activates mast cells, which release their granules of histamine. The flood of histamine irritates the nasal lining and triggers mucus production and then a sneeze, as well as activating your tear glands. Luckily your hay fever is mild, and other immune system cells release soothing signaling chemicals that suppress the activity of the mast cells and the B cells that make IgE.

Shower power

Studies have shown that taking regular cold showers or baths can reduce your chances of catching a cold. If this sounds too painful, try turning your shower to cold for a few seconds just before you get out—this will stimulate the movement of blood through your system.

8:00 P.M. Down and dirty

A tackle during your weekly soccer game sends you sprawling in the mud, and dirt gets into the cut on your hand. Soil bacteria now find themselves in a richly nutritious environment, but your immune defenses quickly swing into action. Your wound is already full of neutrophils and monocytes—between them they make short work of the invading microbes. Neutrophils bathe them in corrosive enzymes, and the monocytes consume them and display their antigens to other immune system cells. The monocytes also release chemotaxins, signaling substances that attract other cells to the area, particularly fibroblasts, which make scar tissue, blocking off the wound and preventing more bacteria from getting in.

6:00 P.M. Vacation shot

After work, you keep your appointment at the doctor's office, where you receive the first of the vaccinations needed for your upcoming vacation. In the days following the injection, the antigenic material that is in the vaccine will stimulate the production of antibodies (protein molecules synthesized in lymphoid tissue) that will fight off illness if you are exposed to antigens belonging to the disease while you are abroad.

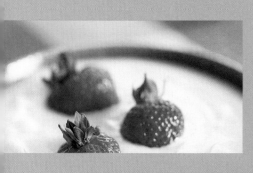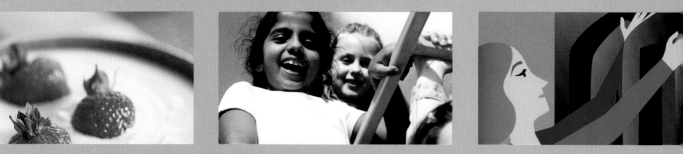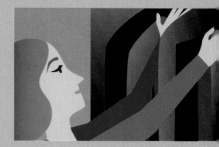

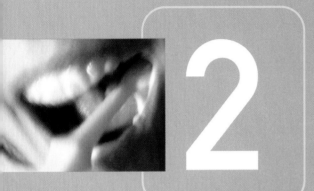

2

Healthy systems for life

TAKE CHARGE OF YOUR HEALTH

The good news about the immune system is that there is a lot you can do on a daily basis to keep it working efficiently so that it can work to protect you from persistent infections, from more serious health problems, and from the potentially harmful effects of the environmental hazards around you.

Prevention is always better than cure, so spotting signs of potential problems early reaps rewards.

Healthy blood can only do its job if the system that pumps it is healthy, too. Keeping blood pressure under control is a key step.

Knowing the risks from the environment and how carcinogens invade the body can help you steer clear of potential health hazards.

Understanding the highly specialized nature of the cells of the immune system can help you support it every day of your life.

When people donate blood, they can be sure that it will be taken safely, analyzed professionally, and used to help others.

Knowing what's normal for you

The signs and symptoms of a blood disorder, or of the immune system not fighting off infection as it should, are often quite subtle. Knowing what is to be expected may help you spot when something is wrong.

The health of your blood and immune system has an enormous impact on your general well-being. Your energy levels and your ability to fight off minor and more serious illnesses depend on the health of your immune system.

NORMAL BLEEDING

The bleeding from minor cuts, such as those from shaving or pricking yourself on a thorn in the garden, should stop fairly quickly. Even a deeper cut should stop bleeding within about seven minutes or so—as long as pressure is applied with a clean cloth. A deep cut may bleed longer; if it soaks through your first cloth, add a second on top (leave the first one in place). Bleeding from a minor cut that takes a long time to clot could signal a problem; you should see your doctor about this.

People who have problems with their blood clotting properly usually notice bleeding from minor injuries in different parts of the body, together with excessive bruising. Women who have periods that are heavier than usual may have a gynecological problem, but, a problem with clotting may also cause excessively heavy periods.

You should consult your doctor about any unexplained bleeding, whether it clots quickly or not.

Bleeding from the ears or nose

Bleeding from an ear is never normal and should be immediately checked by a doctor. Nosebleeds, on the other hand, are usually harmless. However, a nosebleed may require a doctor's attention if

- blood flows from both nostrils;
- blood is also running down the back of the throat;
- bleeding is still going on 30 minutes after it started; or
- the nosebleed recurs over the next few days.

Bleeding from the gums

Bleeding from the gums is not normal beyond a small amount caused by over-enthusiastic brushing of the teeth. More than this is most likely caused by gum disease—generally gingivitis—especially if the gums are swollen, tender, or painful. Anyone who suspects that he or she has gum disease should see a dentist as soon as possible to get any infection cleared up; otherwise the teeth may loosen and fall out or have to be removed by the dentist. Bleeding gums that are painless may be a symptom of a problem with blood failing to clot as it should normally.

HOW EASILY DO YOU BRUISE?

Bruising is caused by bleeding into the tissues under the skin. Some bruising is perfectly normal: for example, after a bump or a fall. People tend to bruise more easily

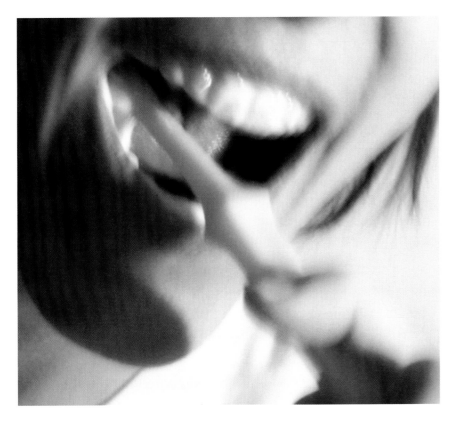

Easy does it
There's a fine line between effective teeth cleaning and over-brushing that causes gums to bleed. If your teeth regularly bleed after brushing, try a softer brush to see if that helps; otherwise, consult a dentist.

HOW TIRED IS TOO TIRED?

Many factors contribute to excessive fatigue—the feeling that you simply can't get out of bed in the morning. In many cases, however, simple lifestyle practices can have an enormous impact on energy levels.

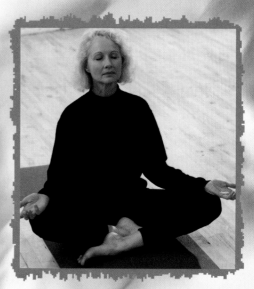

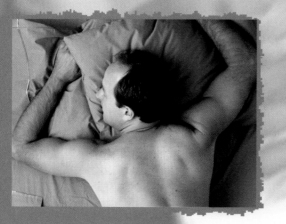

GET ENOUGH SLEEP

Most adults need a minimum of seven hours of quality sleep per night. If you are shortchanging yourself on this, fatigue can build. Keep the bedroom cool and well ventilated and try to establish regular times to go to bed and to get up.

BEAT STRESS AND ANXIETY

Stress is a major cause of fatigue, and worrying about personal problems can exacerbate tiredness. Get help dealing with stress and anxiety, devise a stress management program, or take up meditation, yoga, or tai chi.

as they get older because the tissues under the skin become looser. Those who regularly take steroid drugs may also bruise more easily than normal. A younger person not taking steroid drugs who bruises easily may have a problem with blood clotting that warrants further investigation. Unexplained bruising should be brought to the attention of a doctor, as should any bruise that does not begin to improve within two weeks or has not healed completely within a month.

SWOLLEN LYMPH GLAND

The most common cause of swollen lymph glands is infection. For example, a sore throat caused by a viral infection will cause swelling of the lymph glands in the neck. The glands may be tender to touch. This shouldn't alarm you or cause you to see the doctor. But swollen lymph glands can also be caused by a more serious infection and sometimes by cancer. In this case, the lymph glands all over the body may be swollen or tender, and the swelling will not disappear after a few days, as in normal infections. If you have these symptoms, consult your doctor.

COLD EXTREMITIES

When you go out in cold weather, it is normal for your body to reduce the amount of blood reaching your hands and feet. This is the body's automatic response to cold, designed to protect the vital internal organs, such as the brain, liver, and kidneys. Sometimes you may notice that your hands change color and become numb or even painful. All this can be normal, and it tends to be more common in women than in men.

It is not normal for hands to stay painful for several minutes after they have been warmed up—this may signal Raynaud's phenomenon (see page 151). If your fingers or toes are beginning to show signs of damage from the cold—by developing chilblains, for example—you should seek medical advice.

Prevention is always better than cure with cold extremities: Dress appropriately and try exercises to improve circulation (see pages 76, 77 and 79).

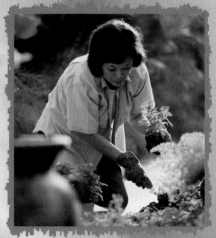

GET SOME EXERCISE
Paradoxically, exercise makes you less—rather than more—tired. Try to build regular exercise, ideally in the fresh air, into your daily life. It does not have to be a sports activity—30 minutes of gardening still counts as exercise.

DRINK SMART
Caffeine is often used for a quick lift, but it stays in the bloodstream for up to eight hours. If you are not sleeping well, avoid tea or coffee after lunchtime. Alcohol can also interrupt sleep patterns. Instead of drinking alcohol, drink plenty of water throughout the day.

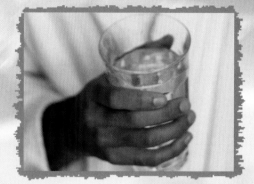

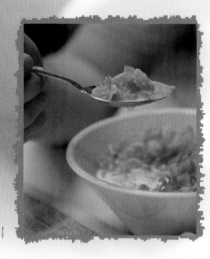

EAT WELL
Have a sizable, fiber-rich breakfast to give you the energy to start the day; then eat regular high-carbohydrate meals and snacks. Avoid high-fat, high-sugar foods that may make you feel energized in the short term, but will lead to sluggishness when their "buzz" wears off.

INFECTIONS IN CHILDREN
It is normal for children to pick up frequent infections, from babyhood on. This is because they have not yet been exposed to most microorganisms and are only gradually building up their immunity. However, if your child is spending more time with a runny nose or sore throat than without, it may be a good idea to consult your doctor, just in case the child's immune system is not functioning as it should be. This is especially true if a child is not growing or putting on weight as expected or if his or her mental development appears to be slightly delayed.

A child who is suffering from a particularly severe infection should see a doctor, especially if there is fever or a rash, or the child is noticeably more quiet and subdued than normal.

INFECTIONS IN ADULTS
The process of catching infections and building up immunity continues throughout adult life. Sometimes a virus will lie dormant in our bodies and become active later; this is normal. One example of this is the chicken pox virus, which can become active as shingles (more than two attacks of shingles a year may mean a problem with the immune system).

GETTING TIRED
It can be very difficult to figure out whether tiredness is normal or not.

Most of us feel tired some of the time, especially when we're bringing up children as well as working hard outside the home. However, if you feel tired after several nights of eight hours of uninterrupted sleep, there may be a problem.

If you have to nap for a few minutes during the day or if doing routine tasks makes you exhausted, you may be suffering from excessive fatigue. Keeping a journal of how tired you are and what makes you feel extra tired can help clarify the issue in your mind. It may also help convince your doctor that something is wrong. Excessive fatigue can be caused by problems such as anemia, an underactive thyroid gland, infection, or chronic fatigue syndrome (see page 140).

Someone becomes anemic when there is a shortage of oxygen-carrying hemoglobin in the blood, which means that tissues throughout the body become deprived of the oxygen they need in order to function effectively. The chief symptom is usually fatigue, regardless of how much sleep you are getting.

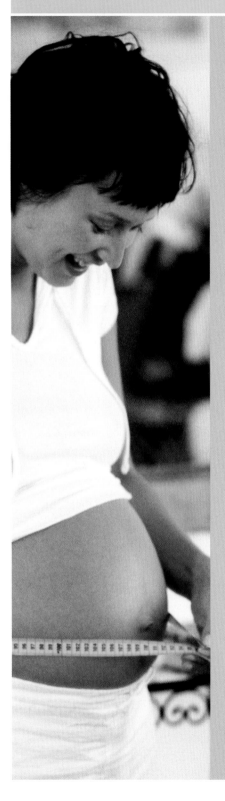

Anemia is a symptom rather than a condition, so diagnosing someone as anemic will prompt further investigations into his or her state of health.

The only way to confirm a case of anemia is to have a complete blood count (see page 105). This will check whether your hemoglobin is at the right level for your age and gender. It is sensible to have this test if you have symptoms that suggest anemia (see page 134), particularly excessive fatigue, or if you have a condition that may cause anemia.

A complete blood count can also provide information on the cause of anemia. For example, if the red blood cells in the sample are unusually small, this shows a deficiency in iron. A patient will then be asked whether he or she has experienced excessive bleeding, and his or her diet will be assessed. The treatment for anemia caused by iron deficiency is a simple and effective course of iron tablets.

Can pregnancy make a woman anemic?

Pregnancy increases the risk of anemia because there is an increase in demand for iron and other vitamins. The iron needed to make hemoglobin in the blood is distributed to both the mother and her baby. This results in the woman's own iron levels being reduced, leading to anemia. Iron can easily be replaced by supplements or changes in diet. Folic acid is another key component of hemoglobin, and a deficiency can also lead to anemia.

Can losing blood cause anemia?

Excessive bleeding (heavy periods or blood loss during surgery) can cause anemia by depleting the body's stores of iron. Small cuts, such as those you can get while cooking, will not cause anemia.

What are the signs or symptoms to look out for?

The main symptoms of iron deficiency anemia are very pale skin, an increase in the number of minor infections, weakness, fatigue, tiredness, and breathlessness on slight exertion.

Can lifestyle affect iron levels?

An imbalanced diet can lead to iron deficiency.

Is it possible to eat a good, balanced diet and still suffer from low iron levels and anemia?

Nutrients can be poorly absorbed because of a disorder or disease of the digestive system, leading to deficiencies that can cause anemia. For example, pernicious anemia (see page 151) is caused by cells that help absorb vitamin B_{12} having been damaged by the immune system, leading to vitamin B_{12} deficiency.

Can anemia be a symptom of more serious conditions?

Blood diseases such as leukemia also cause anemia.

Keeping blood pressure under control

High blood pressure, or hypertension, is a common condition that over time can damage the arteries, brain, kidneys, and heart. The consequences of uncontrolled hypertension include coronary artery disease and strokes.

The majority of cases of high blood pressure (hypertension) are not caused by any particular disease. Instead, people with high blood pressure tend to fall into at least one of the following categories.

- They have a family history of high blood pressure.
- They tend to eat a lot of salt.
- They are overweight.
- They do not get much exercise.
- They experience high stress levels.
- They drink alcohol in excess.
- They smoke.

Relatively rarely, hypertension may be caused by diseases that affect organs such as the kidneys and adrenal glands (which secrete blood pressure controlling hormones).

BLOOD PRESSURE CHECKS

- Healthy people under age 45 should have their blood pressure checked every two years. Because hypertension may cause no noticeable symptoms, having a regular check is an easy way to pick up any unhealthy rise in blood pressure before the complications of hypertension develop.
- People at risk for hypertension because of family history or lifestyle should have their blood pressure measured more frequently —at least once a year, sometimes more—as should those who have a family history of heart disease or problems with the blood vessels, kidneys, or endocrine system.

- Pregnant women should have their blood pressure checked at each checkup, because high blood pressure can be dangerous for both mother and baby.

Although you can buy blood pressure measuring devices, it's best to have blood pressure measured by a medical professional who is trained in the technique and will use equipment that is checked for accuracy.

For some people, the stress of just visiting the doctor can push up their blood pressure (so-called white-coat hypertension). If your blood pressure is high on a single occasion, a second test will be arranged; try to make sure you are able to rest and relax for a few minutes before the test. If you have hypertension, your doctor may set up urine and blood tests to rule out underlying diseases. There may also be tests such as a heart trace to check for complications from the hypertension.

NORMAL BLOOD PRESSURE

There are two parts to the measurement of blood pressure. The first is the systolic reading, taken as the heart beats, and the second is the diastolic reading, taken as the heart muscle relaxes again.

Blood pressure varies enormously from individual to individual and over time. There are some general guidelines, however.

- A healthy blood pressure is a systolic reading of less than 130 and a diastolic reading of less than 85 (this will be expressed as 130/85).

- Your doctor may recommend lifestyle changes if your blood pressure reaches 140/90.
- Medication will probably be prescribed when blood pressure reaches 160/100. An individual with blood pressure at this level is not considered a good candidate for surgery, so medication to lower it and keep it down will be needed if any surgery is planned.

Try to keep calm during a test
Blood pressure measurements vary throughout the day depending on activity level and even your emotional state. Blood pressure is lower during periods of sleep and usually rises in response to exercise.

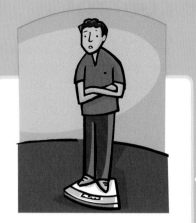

Weight control
Keep your weight within the healthy weight range for your height and gender.

Stress buster
Find some practical ways for managing stress and put them into practice.

Salt alert
Reduce your salt intake—this may require advice from a dietitian, but a simple effective strategy is to cut down on processed foods and snacks. Experts suggest limiting daily intake to about 5g —a slightly heaped teaspoon.

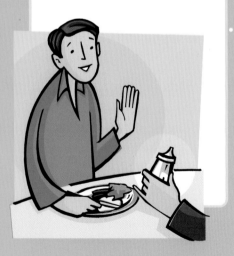

WHAT YOU CAN DO TO KEEP BLOOD PRESSURE WITHIN HEALTHY LIMITS

There is good evidence that anti-hypertensive drugs control blood pressure and reduce the risk of the side effects of hypertension. But other than drugs, there is a lot that you can do to treat your own hypertension or to reduce the chances of developing hypertension in the first place.

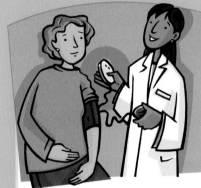

Know the risks
Hypertension runs in families, so if your parents suffered, you might, too. Have your blood pressure checked regularly, particularly if you are over age 45.

Limit alcohol intake
Keep your alcohol intake within guidelines—if you want to control your blood pressure you probably shouldn't drink more than a glass of wine a day, with some alcohol-free days each week.

Get moving
Get 30 minutes of brisk exercise three times a week. This does not mean going to the gym if you don't want to: Walking and gardening are both good forms of exercise.

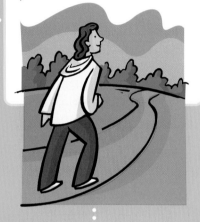

Eat smart
Reducing fat and increasing fiber won't directly help your blood pressure, but it will reduce the risk of heart attacks.

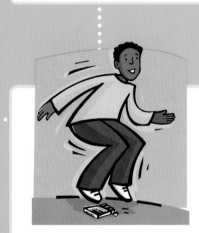

Quit smoking
Smoking is a major contributor to high blood pressure. Use every available resource to stop smoking cigarettes.

Be aware of risk factors

The world around us contains many threats to the health of our blood and lymph systems. General pollutants can contaminate air, water, or soil, and smoking and drinking too much alcohol can affect others as well as ourselves.

Chemicals, bacteria, viruses, drugs, and toxins can all trigger problems in the immune system.

CARCINOGENS

Carcinogens are substances that increase the risk of cancer developing, usually by causing damage to the DNA within cell nuclei. Some scientists suggest that carcinogens clear the way for cancer cells to appear and multiply by damaging the immune system. This is a possibile —not the usual—cause of cancer. Patients with severely damaged immune systems—resulting from HIV or immunosuppressive drugs, for example—are at higher risk of developing cancer than other people. Conversely, only a few cancers, such as lymphoma (see page 150), myeloma (see page 150), and chronic lymphatic leukemia (see page 148) cause significant damage to the immune system.

Cigarette smoking

Cigarette smoke is a potent carcinogen. One in ten smokers will develop cancer of the lungs, tongue, stomach, or bladder. Smoking also causes cancer of the kidney, pancreas, liver, and nose, as well as leukemia.

Alcohol

Alcohol is a carcinogen linked to cancer of the esophagus and breast. In addition, alcohol decreases levels of zinc, which is essential to the healthy functioning of the immune system. However, moderate drinking —say one drink a day, particularly a glass of red wine with a meal—can actually improve your state of health.

Medicines

All medicinal drugs are thoroughly tested for carcinogenicity before they become available to patients. Some types of chemotherapy, used to treat cancer, do increase the risk of another cancer developing several years later. However, potential risks are always carefully assessed before treatment starts. More often, bone marrow failure (see page 138) is a consequence of taking these drugs.

EXTERNAL THREATS

The world around us can also have an enormous impact on health. There are many things we can do to reduce potential risks.

Lead poisoning

Taking in too much lead poses a particular threat to children, who are more likely than adults to suffer ill-effects. Lead poisoning can cause a type of anemia and brain damage.

FOR BABIES

Protecting babies from lead in tap water

Bottle-fed babies are at risk of lead poisoning if the tap water that is added to their formula has any lead in it. So, too, are babies who drink water or juice mixed with water, even if they are mainly breastfed. Boiling drinking water may kill bacteria, but it does not get rid of the lead content. There are ways to protect your baby.

- If there is reason to suspect that the water in your home is passing through lead piping (as in many older buildings) or that a leaded solder has been used to seal water pipe joints (as is done illegally in some new houses), get the lead levels tested by the local authority or water company. If levels are high, the cause should be established and any affected piping or solder replaced.

- Wherever you are, only take drinking water from the cold water tap in the kitchen. Let the faucet run for at least a minute before taking any water. If in doubt, prepare formula or food from bottled water.

MINIMIZING YOUR RISKS

There is a lot you can do to limit your exposure to potential threats and in some cases to remove them altogether from your environment.

Have any lead pipes in your house replaced; if you are unsure, the local water company or Environmental Protection Agency can detail what to look for.

In a house built before 1970, make sure all flaking paint is well sealed.

The risk to health of radiation from radon, naturally emitted from granite rocks, is tiny...

... But if your home is on granite, it can be tested for radon, and you can get advice on sealing the ground floor and on ventilation.

There is little evidence that cellular phones are harmful to health, but little that they are safe, either. The government recommends limiting children's use of them.

Lead poisoning is less of a threat than it once was because it has been withdrawn from gasoline and paints no longer contain lead. Lead-contaminated drinking water may be a problem in buildings with lead in the plumbing system.

Radiation

There are many forms of radiation, including ionizing radiation (X-rays and rays from nuclear reactions), electromagnetic radiation (from electrical currents), and microwaves (from cell phones, for example). Like chemical carcinogens, radiation can cause cancer by damaging the DNA within cells.

There is no doubt that large, concentrated doses of radiation are harmful. However, there is as yet little evidence of an increased incidence of blood disorders, cancer, or problems with the immune system in those who have been exposed to ionizing radiation accidentally released into the atmosphere.

There is much controversy surrounding the effects of nuclear power plants on health, particularly cancer. Studies in both the U.S. and the UK have shown that workers do not have an increased incidence of cancer when compared with the general population. There has also been concern that people living in the area of nuclear plants may have been exposed to long-term higher levels of radiation. Some research has shown that these people have an increased risk of developing cancer.

Other studies have revealed that levels of certain cancers, particularly those of blood and bone, in children living in the area of nuclear plants are higher than the national average. It has been suggested this may be caused by fathers of affected children

having been damaged by radiation, but research has not revealed any direct evidence to support this. A theory about a nuclear plant in England suggests that the many "outsiders" who moved into the area to work at the plant in the 1950s naturally brought all sorts of viruses with them and that this increased leukemia and lymphoma levels.

Gulf War syndrome

During the Gulf War of 1991, troops were exposed to many chemicals and pollutants. Pesticides were used extensively. The many oil well fires exposed soldiers to pollutants caused by petroleum combustion. Drinking water was contaminated or over-chlorinated and vehicles were sprayed with camouflage paint. Soldiers were also given vaccines designed to protect them from disease and from chemical attack.

After the war, thousands of veterans suffered a variety of symptoms—including fatigue, joint pain, skin problems, depression, and memory loss—called Gulf War syndrome. Lawyers acting for some soldiers have suggested that the chemicals to which they were exposed may have damaged their nervous systems or that the multiple vaccines may have overstimulated or exhausted their immune systems, leading to their health problems. So far, however, scientists have not confirmed a definite link between Gulf War syndrome and either vaccines or chemicals.

A healthy immune system

The immune system fights off infection, which involves eliminating anything foreign to the body. It also remembers what it has met before; this allows a vigorous response when a foreign body is encountered for the second time.

The body's war against infection is fought by cells and proteins carried in body fluids. Key players include

- phagocytes,
- complement proteins,
- T cells, and
- antibodies.

The role of phagocytes

Phagocytes are cells in our bodily fluids that track down and engulf microorganisms such as bacteria and fungi. The name phagocyte comes from the Greek words meaning "eating cells." Without phagocytes our bodies would be overwhelmed by infection. If not treated, a patient who develops neutropenia—a deficiency of phagocytes—would probably die of infection within just a few hours.

The role of complement proteins

Invading microorganisms that are too fast for the phagocytes are attacked by a group of proteins called complement proteins. These can be found at any place in the body where a foreign cell can gain access and cause infection, such as the mucous membranes lining the mouth or gastrointestinal tract. Just a few bacteria can activate millions of complement proteins, and the complement proteins attract phagocytes to the site of infection to finish the job of destroying invading microorganisms.

T cells versus viruses

Viruses can only live and reproduce inside cells, and they are totally dependent on the host cell's machinery for all their needs. Living only inside cells means they cannot be identified as invaders by that body's phagocytes and complement proteins. It is likely that the T cell evolved to overcome this problem: It is T cells that detect and kill cells infected with viruses.

Antibodies and allergic reactions

Antibodies are special kinds of proteins that help the immune system recognize, target, and attack any substance that the body regards as foreign or possibly dangerous (see page 36). They are produced by a type of white blood cell called B cells. Any substance that provokes an attack from an antibody is known as an antigen.

Antibodies normally react to and destroy antigens in your body without you experiencing any side effects. Sometimes, however, certain antigens cause the body to overreact.

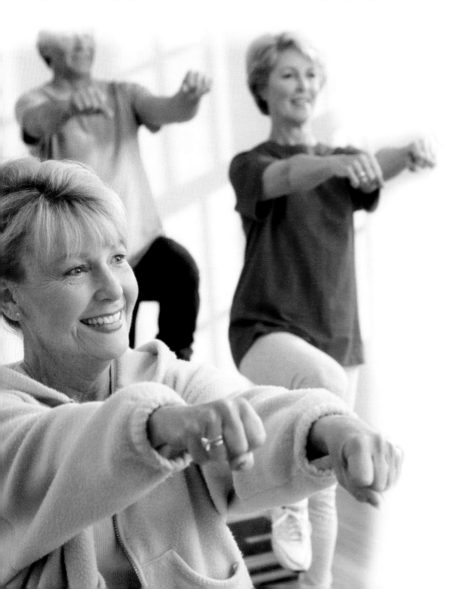

Keep it moderate
Regular exercise improves blood circulation and boosts the speed with which the immune system responds to invaders. Some studies have shown light to moderate exercise to be more beneficial than more intense workouts.

51

FOR BABIES

Breastfeeding and the immune system

Unborn babies are connected to their mothers by the placenta. The IgG class of antibody travels from the mother, through the placenta, and into the unborn baby, so that at birth, the baby has some immunity to infection (a child's own immune system is not mature until about age five). After birth, a mother passes antibodies of the IgA class to her baby in her breast milk. Breast milk contains antibodies to fight every infection to which the mother has been exposed. Together, the IgG and IgA antibodies give breastfed babies greater levels of immunity. This method of passing on immunity is shared by all mammals, who feed their babies on milk.

Whenever these particular antigens (called allergens) are encountered, a type of antibody called IgE provokes a dramatic response as the body tries to expel the allergen. The classic example is hay fever, in which IgE antibodies trigger the expulsion of the pollen allergen through a runny nose and sneezing. This type of overreaction is referred to as hypersensitivity.

Fighting the common cold

The reason that a cold usually lasts only three or four days is because T cells clear the virus that caused it. In the process of killing the virus, T cells divide many times, and by the end of the process, there will be several million of them capable of recognizing that specific cold virus. Some of these T cells survive for many years. This means that if you are exposed to the same virus again, your immune system will respond more quickly and you will not suffer a full-blown cold from that virus again. Unfortunately, there are many different strains of cold virus, which is why we keep catching colds.

WHEN THE IMMUNE SYSTEM TURNS ON ITSELF

The vast majority of immune responses are helpful, enabling our bodies to eliminate infections and cancerous cells. Almost all T cells and antibodies are conditioned not to attack any cells produced by the host's own body. For T cells, this conditioning takes place within the thymus (an organ just behind the breast bone); for antibodies, it happens in the bone marrow.

Inevitably, however, the body does produce some T cells and antibodies that target harmless cells belonging to the host's own body. The immune system gets around this by ordering these autoimmune T and B cells to self-destruct.

However, antibodies and T cells do sometimes attack the body's own tissues, giving rise to a variety of disorders loosely called "autoimmune diseases." Perhaps the best-known examples of autoimmune diseases are pernicious anemia, rheumatic fever, rheumatoid arthritis, and SLE (systemic lupus erythematosus).

IMMUNOLOGICAL MEMORY

The body's ability to defend itself against invaders such as bacteria and viruses is called immunity. The human immune system can remember most invaders it has encountered before: A second encounter with the same agent prompts a rapid immune response. This is called immunological memory, and it means that an individual basically becomes immune to a particular toxin.

Immunization and vaccines

By taking advantage of immunological memory, vaccines do not need to contain live, potentially dangerous microorganisms. Instead, they utilize proteins from microorganisms to stimulate immunological memory. Vaccines are the major immunological success story of the last century and have saved hundreds of millions of lives (see pages 88–91).

UNDERSTANDING THREATS TO YOUR IMMUNE SYSTEM

The immune system is integral to the efficient functioning of every part of your body—even your brain. If you are suffering from an infection, for example, the immune system instructs the brain to raise your body temperature in an attempt to destroy the invading organism; this is why fever is such a classic symptom of infection. In addition, when you have a fever, the immune system directs the brain to make you feel tired so that you will sleep more and reduces your appetite so that you eat less.

Conversely, many behaviors, disorders, and medical treatments that affect your various body systems will also affect the immune system.

- Any kind of stress will have negative effects on the immune system. Experiments have shown that even a short stressful stimulus, such as a loud noise, sends signals to the brain and endocrine glands and has a measurable negative effect on the immune system. More prolonged stress has more serious effects. For example, the psychological stress of bereavement can weaken the immune system.
- Excessive exercise may weaken the immune system. Athletes suffer more coughs and colds while training for competitions than at other times. This is one reason why exercise has to be balanced and why it is not good to push yourself too hard (see pages 84–85).
- Repeated use of some drugs to treat infections—notably steroids and broad-spectrum antibiotics—can destroy beneficial bacteria in the gastrointestinal tract; these bacteria play an important role in the functioning of the immune system. Probiotics can help restore the balance.
- Areas of localized infection—such as dental abcesses or infected tonsils—may disturb the normal immune system processes of neutralizing and eliminating an infection.
- When you cough, you are clearing the airways and lungs of infected matter. Cough suppression medications block this natural process, so infection is not expelled as it should be, and the efficiency of the immune system is consequently lowered.
- People who take large quantities of herbs need to know about possible side effects—for example, large quantities of licorice can lead to salt retention and high blood pressure. Many experts believe that relaxation techniques are a safer and more effective complementary therapy for the immune system.

Herbs that may boost the immune system

Many people take herbs for an immune system boost and often feel better for it, but no herb should be taken in excess.

Astragalus root *(Astragalus membranaceus)*
Some people believe that Chinese astragalus root—also known as milk vetch—is a powerful stimulator of the immune system in general. It is often used to ward off or treat the common cold.

Echinacea *(Echinacea angustifolia)*
This wildflower from North America, the coneflower, is thought to be one of the most effective and popular enhancers of the immune system used in the West. It is believed to trigger resistance against colds, the flu, and many other infections.

Usnea *(Usnea barbata)*
A common lichen, usnea is an immune system tonic that targets bacterial infections, but it may be of overall benefit whenever the body is fighting infection.

Poke root *(Phytolacca americana)*
Herbalists believe that poke root tincture is best used to counter infections centered in the throat, chest, and lungs. It works well when taken with echinacea.

Ginseng root *(Panax ginseng)*
As well as stimulating nonspecific resistance to infection, this Chinese herb has traditionally been used to help the body fight fatigue and stress (though there is little scientific evidence of its effectiveness as an energy booster).

Garlic *(Allium sativum)*
Garlic is an antiseptic and blood cleanser, good for mucus-producing infections. Tablets made from freeze-dried garlic do not cause the breath problems associated with fresh garlic.

Licorice *(Glycyrrhiza glabra)*
This herb helps the immune system by stimulating the formation of white blood cells and antibodies. In particular, it fights infection within the respiratory tract. It also stimulates production of energy-boosting epinephrine.

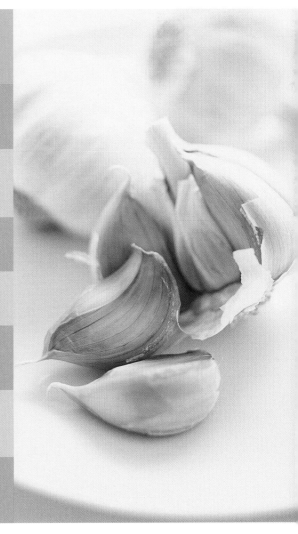

LIFESTYLE SUPPORT FOR THE IMMUNE SYSTEM

In addition to avoiding behaviors that increase your susceptibility to infection, you can also take various positive measures to strengthen your immune system's response to infection.

EAT A BALANCED DIET

A balanced diet is just one important contribution you can make to ensure that you have a healthy immune system. To make sure you have a good balance of vitamins and minerals, including micronutrients such as zinc, eat a mixed diet that is low in fat, with adequate amounts of protein and carbohydrates and plenty of fruit and vegetables. This should keep the immune system in good condition without relying on dietary additives or supplements. In fact, some nutrients—such as vitamin D—can damage your immune system and other body systems if taken in excess.

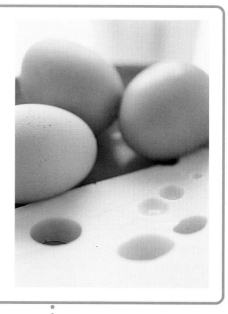

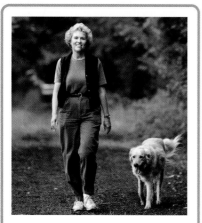

RELAX—DON'T DO IT

Stress is known to hinder the immune system, so learning to relax should improve its functioning—even though there is no hard evidence of this from clinical trials. Take time to find a way of relaxing that works for you. This could be anything from yoga to a gentle walk in the park with the dog.

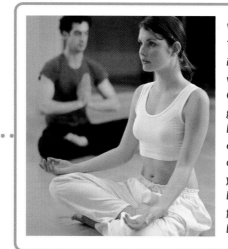

VISUALIZATION TECHNIQUES

The power of the mind can bolster the immune system by means of "creative visualization" or "guided imagery." Concentrating on relaxing images is a good way to reduce stress levels, which benefits the immune system. Scientific evidence is lacking, however, on whether or not focusing your thoughts on boosting your body's defenses—visualizing a virus being chased out of your bloodstream, for example—can really improve your body's ability to resist infection.

HYDROTHERAPY

Research has shown that regular cold baths or showers and swimming in cold water have a stimulating effect on the immune system. One study that compared university students who had a daily cold bath with those who did not showed that the cold bath takers suffered from significantly fewer colds.

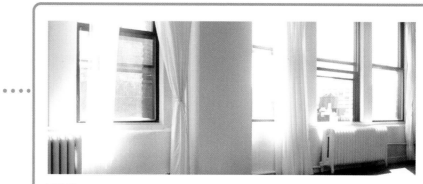

LIGHT

There is some evidence that people who live and work in artificial light have more infections that those who experience lots of daylight, pointing to the importance of sunlight to the immune system.

Why give blood?

American hospitals use 32,000 pints of donated blood every day. One person needs blood every three seconds. Although about 60 percent of the U.S. population is eligible to donate, only 5 percent does, leading to frequent shortages.

WHAT HAPPENS WHEN YOU GIVE BLOOD?

In the United States, blood donation is entirely voluntary. The American Red Cross and other collection centers operate a donor selection policy that protects the health of both the blood donor and the recipient. There are strict donor selection guidelines. Donors are asked to provide a form of identification before each donation; after the first time, this can be your Red Cross donor card. Donors are asked to fill out a donor questionnaire and to answer pertinent questions, in private, relating to their health. When there is concern for the health of a donor or potential recipient, the donor may be permanently excluded or deferred for a defined period. A short term deferral can occur if you are anemic or have a cold or the flu on collection day.

The ideal donor will be at least 17 years old, weigh at least 110 pounds, and be in good health. Each donated pint of blood is subjected to up to 12 tests, including those for HIV, hepatitis B and C, and syphilis. The following guidelines are occasionally revised and may vary depending on the blood bank. Donors are permanently excluded if

- they are HIV positive;
- they are hepatitis B or C carriers;
- they are at increased risk of Creutzfeldt-Jakob Disease (CJD);
- they have sickle cell disease.

Donors are deferred for 12 months if

- they engage in behavior that puts them at increased risk for contracting HIV/AIDS or hepatitis;
- they are being treated for syphilis or gonorrhea;

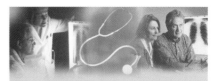

Milestones
IN MEDICINE

In 1901, Karl Landsteiner discovered the first human blood group system, which he called the ABO system. He defined four basic groups within this system: A, B, AB, and O. "Landsteiner's law" was based on the discovery that blood clumping, or agglutination, occurs during a transfusion when the recipient carries antibodies against the donor blood cells. Specifically, the plasma of a person contains natural antibodies to A or B if those antigens are absent from that person's red cells.

- they recently had an organ or tissue transplant or received a blood trnasfusion;
- they have recently visited a malarial area (the deferment lasts for 3 years if the donor has moved from an area where malaria is found or if the donor was treated for malaria);
- they have had any part of their body pierced or gotten a tattoo in the last year.

About 45 percent of Americans have type O blood, 40 percent have type A, 10 percent have type B, and 5 percent are AB; 85 percent of the population is Rh positive.

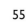

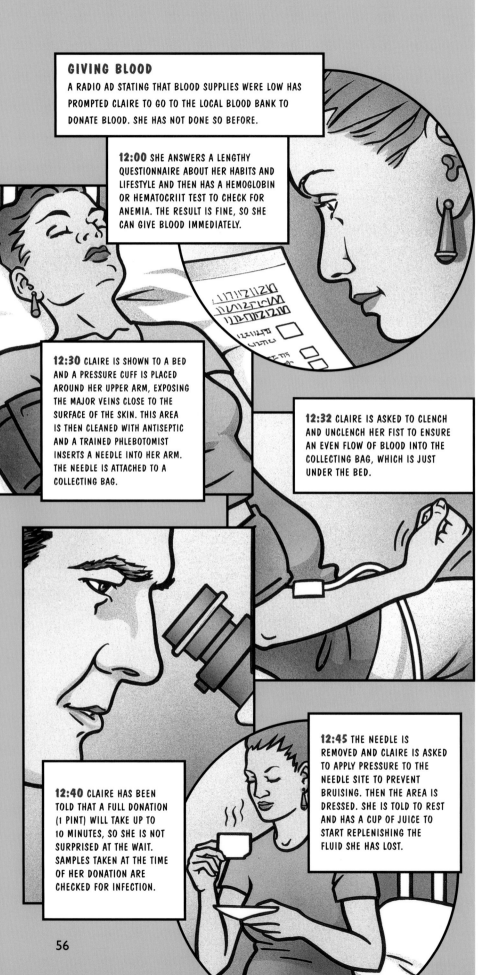

GIVING BLOOD

A RADIO AD STATING THAT BLOOD SUPPLIES WERE LOW HAS PROMPTED CLAIRE TO GO TO THE LOCAL BLOOD BANK TO DONATE BLOOD. SHE HAS NOT DONE SO BEFORE.

12:00 SHE ANSWERS A LENGTHY QUESTIONNAIRE ABOUT HER HABITS AND LIFESTYLE AND THEN HAS A HEMOGLOBIN OR HEMATOCRIIT TEST TO CHECK FOR ANEMIA. THE RESULT IS FINE, SO SHE CAN GIVE BLOOD IMMEDIATELY.

12:30 CLAIRE IS SHOWN TO A BED AND A PRESSURE CUFF IS PLACED AROUND HER UPPER ARM, EXPOSING THE MAJOR VEINS CLOSE TO THE SURFACE OF THE SKIN. THIS AREA IS THEN CLEANED WITH ANTISEPTIC AND A TRAINED PHLEBOTOMIST INSERTS A NEEDLE INTO HER ARM. THE NEEDLE IS ATTACHED TO A COLLECTING BAG.

12:32 CLAIRE IS ASKED TO CLENCH AND UNCLENCH HER FIST TO ENSURE AN EVEN FLOW OF BLOOD INTO THE COLLECTING BAG, WHICH IS JUST UNDER THE BED.

12:40 CLAIRE HAS BEEN TOLD THAT A FULL DONATION (1 PINT) WILL TAKE UP TO 10 MINUTES, SO SHE IS NOT SURPRISED AT THE WAIT. SAMPLES TAKEN AT THE TIME OF HER DONATION ARE CHECKED FOR INFECTION.

12:45 THE NEEDLE IS REMOVED AND CLAIRE IS ASKED TO APPLY PRESSURE TO THE NEEDLE SITE TO PREVENT BRUISING. THEN THE AREA IS DRESSED. SHE IS TOLD TO REST AND HAS A CUP OF JUICE TO START REPLENISHING THE FLUID SHE HAS LOST.

People in this deferred group will have had a clearly identified episode of risk, but the overall risk of them having an infection that is transmissible by blood transfusion is low. The 12 months act as a period of quarantine, giving time for evidence of infection or a positive test result to appear.

Donors are sometimes deferred for a given period, usually short, if

- they are pregnant;
- they have had recent complicated dental work;
- they are currently on medication (depending on the medication);
- they have had contact with an infectious disease or have recently had certain immunizations such as hepatitis B or small pox.

The donor's specific eligibility will be assessed before donation. Call the American Red Cross at 1-800-GIVE-LIFE to learn more about your eligibility.

At a single donor session, about 0.8–1 pint of blood is taken. The average woman has 8 pints of blood and the average man has 10 pints, so no more than 10 percent of the total blood volume is taken in a donation.

Feeling faint

Some people feel faint after giving blood, so it is important to follow all the advice given after the donation. Donors should replenish lost fluid by drinking plenty, but they must avoid alcohol. Smoking should also be avoided because the effects of nicotine will be much stronger after giving blood. It is important not to rush around—however, do not stand or sit still for long periods of time because this can lead to blood pooling in the legs. If you do feel faint, bend forward with your head between your knees; when you feel ready to get up move slowly, but if you still feel faint, lie down.

WHAT ARE THE RISKS OF GIVING BLOOD?

Blood donation is very safe and in fact, most donors feel better for having given a pint of blood. Donating blood could theoretically make you anemic, but your hemoglobin level will be carefully checked before each donation.

Some people worry that they might catch infections from donating blood, but the equipment used (needles, tubing) is in sterile condition and will not have been used before. The chances of catching an infection are close to zero.

STORING BLOOD

Blood is separated into its components when it is taken: red blood cells, platelets, and plasma. The components are labeled with the blood type and stored at appropriate temperatures—plasma, for example, can be frozen and will last longer.

PLATELETS

Platelets are the smallest of the blood cells, and they play an important role in hemostasis, clumping together to form a physical barrier to prevent blood loss. Patients with a low platelet count are prone to bruising and internal bleeding, and in severe cases, they can literally bleed to death. Most platelet donations are used to prevent bleeding in patients who are temporarily unable to make their own platelets, such as cancer or leukemia patients or patients with an autoimmune disease in which platelets are destroyed by the patient's own immune system. It is usual for patients to receive so-called "whole blood donations," in which

Identical twins are the only people who will have the same antigens on their red blood cells.

platelets from three different donations are pooled into one pack. Patients who require chronic platelet support are given the same number of platelets from just one donor.

THE ABO BLOOD GROUPS

There are a number of systems for identifying different blood groups. The ABO system is the best known and the most important when it comes to giving blood. Within this system, each person's blood type is determined genetically, and whether you are type A, B, AB, or O will depend on the blood types of your parents. In each case, the major differences depend on the presence (or lack) of certain protein molecules in the blood, specifically antigens—found on the surface of the red blood cells—and antibodies found in blood plasma.

ABO incompatibility

Not all blood types are compatible, and mixing them can lead to blood clumping or agglutination. A person will typically develop antibodies to the antigens that are missing. So, if a person has type A antigens on the surface of his or her red blood cells, he or she will have B antibodies (anti-B agglutins) in his or her blood plasma. If he or she receives a type-B blood transfusion, the antibodies will start to destroy the transfused red cells, possibly with fatal consequences. This is why type A blood must never be given to a type B person.

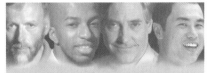

BLOOD GROUPS AND PATERNITY

Because of the frequency of the genes in the population, blood groups cannot be used to prove paternity, but it is possible to use them to disprove paternity.

- Two parents who are A can only have a child who is A or O.
- Two parents who are B can only have a child who is B or O.
- An A parent and a B parent can have a child of any group.
- An A and AB or a B and AB cannot have an O child. Two O parents can only have an O child.

It is possible for two Rhesus (Rh) positive parents to have an Rh negative child, but it is not possible for negative parents to have a positive child. The man, woman, and child must all be tested.

Demonstrating the system

The "tile technique" is used to demonstrate how the system works. The serum from each of blood group A individuals (anti-B), blood group B individuals (anti-A), and blood group O individuals (anti-A and anti-B) is mixed with red cells of unknown ABO blood group. The tile is rocked gently so the serum and the red cells mix. Clumping (agglutination) of the cells occurs where there is an antibody specific to the antigens on the red cells. Each reaction has a specific pattern—this can be clearly identified by the technician. Where there is no antibody–antigen reaction, the red cells remain in suspension.

WHICH BLOOD TYPES ARE COMPATIBLE?

People with type A blood cannot receive type B blood and vice versa.
Those with blood type O are universal donors because there are no antigens to attack.
AB people are the best receivers, because they have no antibodies to other blood types.

BLOOD GROUP	ANTIGENS	ANTIBODIES	CAN GIVE TO	CAN RECEIVE FROM
AB	A and B	None	AB	AB, A, B, O
A	A	B	A and AB	A and O
B	B	A	B and AB	B and O
O	None	A and B	AB, A, B, O	O

ANTIGENS AND AGGLUTINS

A person's blood plasma contains natural antibodies (agglutins) to A or B, if those antigens are absent from that person's red cells.

BLOOD TYPE	ANTIGENS PRESENT	ANTIBODIES PRESENT
AB	AB	None
A	A	Anti-B
B	B	Anti-A
O	None	Anti-A and anti-B

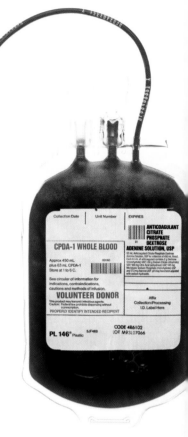

THE RHESUS SYSTEM

Another significant blood system is the Rhesus system, also discovered by Karl Landsteiner (see page 55) in 1940. The system is named after the Rhesus monkeys on which his experiments were carried out. Regardless of which ABO blood type we have, we will each also be either Rhesus, Rh, positive or Rh negative, depending on whether or not the Rhesus antigen is present on the surface of the red blood cells.

A person with Rh positive blood can receive an Rh negative blood transfusion without any problems. However, a person who has Rh negative blood may develop antibodies to Rh positive blood if he or she comes into contact with it. This is of particular significance in and happens most commonly in childbearing women who are Rh negative but may be pregnant with a baby who is Rh positive (inherited from the father).

Rhesus disease

Hemolytic disease of the newborn (HDN) is also known as Rhesus disease, because most cases within the last 50 years have been associated with Rh incompatibility. In the simplest terms, HDN is severe neonatal jaundice of unknown cause in succeeding infants born to the same woman.

How does HDN occur?

It is possible for blood cells of an unborn child to pass into the bloodstream of the mother, usually during the birth process, but also following an abortion or miscarriage. If an Rh negative woman is carrying an Rh positive fetus, a natural rejection process will begin, with the mother producing antibodies to attack the foreign red blood cells. Although a firstborn child is at relatively low risk of being affected by this process of immunization, the risk to an unborn fetus increases with each subsequent pregnancy.

Medication is available to prevent Rhesus disease, and it can be given to Rh negative women with Rh positive partners any time there is a chance that fetal cells may enter the pregnant woman's circulation. Used at the right time, the medication is more than 99 percent effective in the prevention of Rhesus disease. However, it is not effective in preventing the disease from worsening once the initial immunization has taken place.

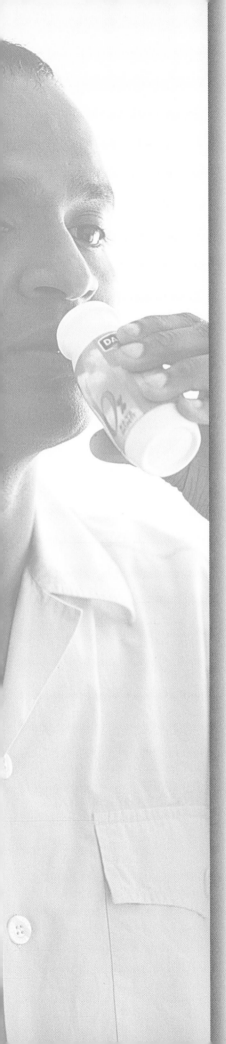

EATING FOR BLOOD AND IMMUNE HEALTH

Eating well is important in keeping every body system, including blood circulation and the immune system, healthy. A balanced and varied diet promotes general health, keeping the blood healthy and enhancing well-being. Understanding the important nutrients and how to get them into your daily diet is a good first step.

 60 *Many vitamins and minerals are involved in working the immune system, and some foods are believed to improve immune function.*

 64 *Delicious drinks and desserts are ideal ways to make sure you get your daily intake of antioxidants from fresh fruits.*

 65 *Keeping up your red blood cell count is vital for health, but many of us—particularly women—do not always get enough iron.*

 70 *In the last 20 years, the vital contribution that folate makes to health—and the effects of too little in the diet—has been recognized.*

 72 *Boosting iron and folate intake is not just about eating liver; simple recipes using varied ingredients make healthy eating a pleasure.*

 74 *Although a little alcohol may be life-enhancing, too much has a serious impact on the blood and immune system.*

59

Boosting the immune system

Many factors are involved in keeping the immune system working well. Some of these are difficult or impossible for an individual to modify, but both stress and diet are under your control and play a central part in your general health.

The efficient functioning of the immune system is influenced by five main factors:

- genetics
- disease
- drugs
- stress
- diet

The body's resistance to infection relies on the immune system. Many factors are involved in keeping the system healthy. You can do nothing about some of them, such as your genes. The factors easiest to modify are stress and diet.

The most important micronutrient for the immune system is zinc. For example, a recent study in an Indian city showed that providing zinc supplements to slum children improved their immunity to infections. Other nutritional factors are probably less important, but it may be worth boosting your intake of antioxidants and probiotics.

Vitamins and minerals involved in immune function include vitamins C, A, E, B_6, folate, and pantothenic acid, essential fatty acids and minerals such as iron, zinc, selenium, calcium, magnesium, manganese, and copper. Some of these are also antioxidants—compounds that help protect your body from damage by free radicals. Free radicals are naturally produced by the body, although sunlight, smoking, and pollution can increase production. There is some evidence that free radicals can damage the immune system, and they also contribute to cancer and arterial disease. If free radicals build up in the body, they can damage our genetic material (DNA), proteins, and polyunsaturated fats. Cells in which the DNA has been damaged are more likely to develop cancer.

In addition, free radicals can play a role in the formation of plaque that can build up on the walls of arteries, eventually causing heart disease. Moreover, the development of cataracts, Alzheimer's disease, physical signs of aging, and inflammation have all been associated with free radical damage. It makes sense for everyone to consume foods and drinks rich in antioxidants to combat free radicals and help protect us from developing diseases of other systems.

The lactose found in fermented milk products like yogurt is much better tolerated than the lactose found in milk.

PROBIOTICS

Technically, a probiotic (from ancient Greek words meaning "for life") is defined by experts as "a live microbial food supplement that beneficially affects the host animal by improving its intestinal microbial balance." In lay terms, this means that if we eat sufficient quantities of beneficial "live" bacteria, we can alter the balance of existing bacteria in the intestine in such a way that the "good/friendly" types of bacteria suppress the growth of disease-causing "bad" bacteria, thereby having positive effects on health.

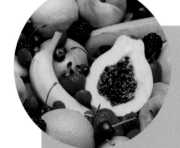

HEALTH-BOOSTING
SUPER NUTRIENTS

Certain vitamins and minerals available in many common foods are particularly beneficial for your general health.

ZINC Found in fortified cereals, seafood, and beef, zinc has been proven to boost the immune system.

VITAMIN E This is present in seeds, vegetable oils, and grains.

CAROTENOIDS Food sources are carrots, melon, red and yellow peppers, mango, spinach, and peaches.

MAGNESIUM Found in oysters, shellfish, herring, liver, legumes, and milk.

VITAMIN C Sources include all fresh fruits, especially citrus fruits and black currants, and vegetables; fruit juices; many other foods are fortified with vitamin C.

SELENIUM This is in oily fish, whole grains, egg yolks, cottage cheese, chicken, sunflower seeds, and garlic.

BIOFLAVONOIDS These can be obtained from fruits and vegetables.

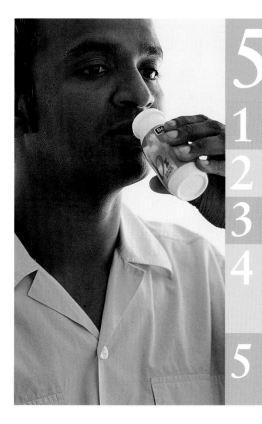

5 Health benefits of lactic acid bacteria

Many people have described the health benefits of lactic acid bacteria, but until recently, these claims were anecdotal. Several studies have now backed up these first findings, and research is ongoing.

1 **IMPROVES LACTOSE ABSORPTION** Lactose is a sugar found in milk and dairy products. Before it can be absorbed into the body, it has to be broken down by an enzyme in the digestive tract called lactase. Undigested lactose causes diarrhea, flatulence, and pain.

2 **HELPS CONSTIPATION** Some studies have shown that among elderly patients, fermented milk products containing lactic acid bacteria help improve the frequency of bowel movements.

3 **PROTECTS AGAINST CANCER** Some studies in animals have suggested that lactic acid bacteria inhibit tumor growth, but evidence among humans is limited.

4 **LOWERS CHOLESTEROL** High levels of low density lipoprotein (LDL)—"bad" cholesterol—in the blood are a known risk factor for heart disease. Some studies have shown that fermented milk products that contain lactic acid bacteria have the ability to lower LDL cholesterol (but this effect could have been caused by the low-fat milk products used rather than the presence of lactic acid bacteria, because low-fat products have cholesterol lowering properties).

5 **IMPROVES IMMUNE FUNCTION** Some animal studies have shown that certain types of lactic acid bacteria stimulate immune function, thereby improving protection against infection and cancer. More studies need to be carried out to confirm these findings.

"Friendly" bacteria have been identified as those that make lactic acid: They include strains of Lactobacillus and Bifidobacterium. If these are present in sufficient numbers in the digestive tract they can help protect us from infection by food-poisoning bacteria such as strains of Salmonella, Shigella, Escherichia, and Clostridium. In addition to producing substances that neutralize toxins, lactic acid bacteria help protect against gastrointestinal infections first by lowering the pH environment of the digestive tract and then by sticking to the surface of the gastrointestinal wall, preventing food-poisoning bacteria from growing and multiplying there.

Products rich in probiotics are readily available in supermarkets and food stores today. The most common of them are flavored drinks based on yogurt or soy that are intended to be consumed daily.

Uncertainties of probiotics

- It is unclear whether probiotics have advantages or disadvantages for children under the age of two because the digestive system is still immature at that age. The effect of changing the balance of the bacteria in the digestive system is unknown.
- It is also unclear whether there is a potential for some strains of probiotic bacteria to transfer antibiotic resistance.

ECHINACEA

Herbalists believe that this plant, native to North America, can boost the immune system, thereby reducing susceptibility to colds and the flu, and help treat yeast, middle ear, respiratory, and urinary tract infections, and to speed the healing of wounds and inflammation. There is not much evidence from clinical trials to support this thinking.

Echinacea is a member of the daisy family, known by many different names including coneflower, Indian head, Kansas snakeroot, sampson root, comb flower, and scurvy root. Three species are used medicinally— *Echinacea angustifolia*, *Echinacea pallida*, and *Echinacea purpurea*. Other species may also be effective, but have not been tried.

Echinacea is available as capsules, dried or fresh herbs, liquid extract, ointment, tablets, teas, and tinctures. Echinacea is not recommended for children, pregnant women, those with autoimmune conditions, or those who are allergic to sunflowers and some other plants such as chrysanthemums. In addition, a course intended to boost the immune system should not last more than four weeks in a row—any longer can lead to suppression of the immune system.

GARLIC

Garlic (*Allium sativum*, literally "all pungent"), is used by herbalists as an antiinflammatory, an immune system stimulant, and an antiviral and antibacterial agent. It is used to treat colds, the flu, infections, heart conditions, and high blood pressure, and is also believed to help prevent atherosclerosis. However, clinical trials have not shown any clear-cut benefits for the immune system.

Garlic is generally available fresh and as capsules, liquid extract, oil, or tincture. It can cause stomachaches in some people. Although most experts agree that garlic is good for you in normal cooking doses, anyone taking anticoagulants is advised to consult a doctor before taking a supplement.

TEA

Tea is rich in flavonoids that act as antioxidants (red wine, nuts, seeds, fruits, and vegetables also contain flavonoids). According to a study looking at flavonoid intake and the long-term risk of heart disease and cancer in seven countries, published in 1995, people who had a higher intake of flavonoids (from onions, red wine, and apples, in addition to

French scientist Louis Pasteur confirmed the antibacterial action of garlic as long ago as 1858.

tea) had a reduced risk of coronary heart disease. Results from long-term studies conducted in the Netherlands and the United States have also supported these findings.

Not all studies have consistently demonstrated this positive effect on health, however. Of the 13 studies published recently, only four have shown a significant relationship between tea drinking and decreased risk of coronary heart disease.

A review looking at the effect of tea drinking and cancer risk published in 2000 reported a number of studies in which green tea was associated with a reduction of risk of cancers of the mouth, esophagus, stomach, colon, rectum, breast, and lung among those drinking five or more cups of tea a day. On the other hand, some studies did not suggest a protective effect of tea against cancer. For example, in the study looking at diet and cancer in the Netherlands, consumption of black tea was not

Leaf of plenty
Tea has been considered as medicine in China for more than 4000 years. Recent studies seem to bear out that tea—especially green tea—may indeed reduce the risk of developing heart disease.

found to affect the risk for stomach, colorectal, lung, and breast cancers.

It is difficult to interpret results from human studies because we have to take into account other lifestyle factors besides the diet, such as whether those studied smoked and their coffee and fat intake. Protective effects could be associated with different lifestyles in different regions of the world. In addition, positive health benefits have mostly been recorded in studies on animals, but the amount of tea drunk by humans is likely to be much less than the doses used to demonstrate disease-preventing effects in a laboratory, so they may not benefit in the same way.

The problem with too much tea

Excessive amounts of tea can interfere with iron absorption from foods such as legumes, grains and vegetables (tea has no effect on the absorption of iron from meat, poultry, or fish) and as such can increase the risk of iron deficiency among vulnerable groups of the population such as infants and toddlers, teenage girls, vegetarians, pregnant women, and the elderly. General advice is to allow at least an hour from the end of a meal before drinking any tea, to minimize any adverse effects on iron absorption.

Tea is good for you

It is clear that tea is a good source of antioxidants, and provided that we keep levels of tea drinking within the guidelines for overall fluid intake of six to eight cups a day, tea can make a positive contribution to health. As an alternative, green tea is known to have higher levels of antioxidants, and studies have shown that it can help lower blood pressure.

EATING MORE IMMUNE-BOOSTING NUTRIENTS

For most people, changes to the diet can improve immune function, as well as contribute to overall health. Variety is key: The more foods you include, the more likely you are to get all the nutrients you need. In some cases, you need only a small amount of a substance to boost the immune system and remain in optimum health.

- Choose fresh whole foods, organic if possible, and cook them as lightly as you can to preserve all their nutrients. B vitamins in particular are depleted by cooking.
- Eat a good selection of raw foods that are packed with vitamins and minerals.
- Include lean red meat in your diet, because it provides iron, selenium, and zinc, which are needed to guard against anemia, as well as helping to heal wounds.

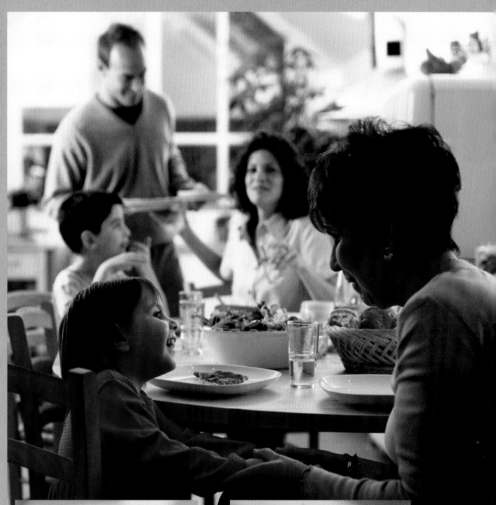

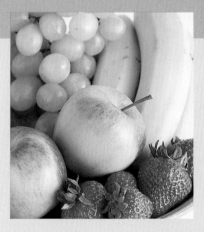

Fruits of plenty
Eat plenty of fruit and vegetables: These will provide antioxidant vitamins A, C, E, folate, and phytochemicals, compounds that are important in protecting against the damaging effects of free radicals on the immune system. Include different-colored fruits and vegetables each day to be sure you fulfill your requirements for different vitamins.

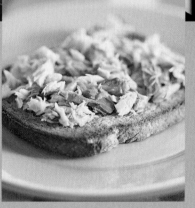

Fish power
Eat more oily fish, which provides essential fatty acids. Essential fatty acids derived from the diet are omega 3 or omega 6 fats, and a deficiency—rare in the Western world—compromises immune function. Try to eat one to two servings of oily fish a week. Vegetables and red meat are also good sources.

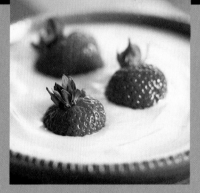

Dairy stars
Include low-fat milk and yogurt in the diet: These will provide calcium and magnesium. Try to avoid dairy products with a high fat content. These can increase the risk of arterial disease.

Health-boosting drinks and desserts

An easy and delicious way to boost your health with food is to increase your intake of fruit. The recipes here are all easy to prepare and take advantage of seasonal and more exotic fruits.

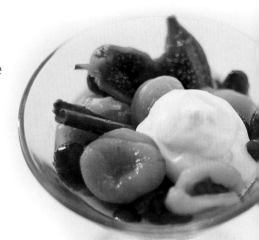

SUMMER BERRIES SALAD

1 lb halved strawberries
1 lb raspberries
1 lb blackberries
½ lb black currants
1 cup elderberry water (made from elderberry liqueur and sparkling water)
1 handful chopped mint, to garnish

Place all the fruits in a large bowl. Pour the elderberry water over them. Chill until ready to serve.
Serves 10–12

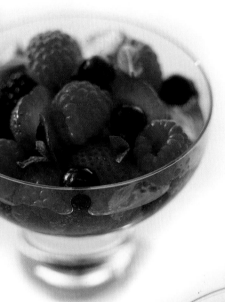

JASMINE-FLAVORED DRIED FRUIT COMPOTE

1 cup water
1 jasmine tea bag
5 oz dried apricots
5 oz dried figs
1½ oz dried cranberries
1 small cinnamon stick
peel of half a lemon
1 tbsp orange blossom honey

Bring the water to boil in a pan, add the tea bag, and simmer for 10 minutes. Remove the bag, add all the other ingredients, and simmer for another 15 minutes until the fruit is tender. Remove the cinnamon stick and lemon peel. Serve chilled with reduced fat yogurt.
Serves 2–3

TROPICAL COOLER

1 ripe papaya, peeled, seeded, chopped
1 cantaloupe, peeled, seeded, chopped
1 ripe mango, peeled, stoned, chopped
sparkling water

Purée the fruit in a blender until smooth. Thin the purée by adding a similar quantity of ice cold sparkling water.
Serves 1–2

BERRY SMOOTHIE

½ cup grape juice
½ cantaloupe, peeled, seeded and chopped
6 ripe strawberries, chopped
4½ oz reduced fat strawberry yogurt

Blend together and serve ice cold.
Serves 1

Foods for healthy blood

What you eat influences the health of your red blood cells, which transport oxygen around your body. Getting enough iron is important, but so is understanding what promotes and prevents efficient iron absorption.

Research suggests that people who get regular intense exercise may need 30 percent more iron than average.

IRON

Iron is a mineral needed for healthy blood. The adult body contains about 4 grams of iron, half of which is found in our red blood cells as hemoglobin, the red pigment. Some iron is present in myoglobin—the protein found in muscle—and the rest is stored in the body's organs.

The primary role of iron as a component of hemoglobin in red blood cells is to transport oxygen from the lungs to the tissues. In addition, iron is required in the makeup of many enzymes needed to perform various functions within the body, such as making steroid hormones and detoxifying foreign compounds in the liver.

A lifetime of iron needs

Iron is not excreted from the body in the urine or through the digestive process; it is lost only with cells from the skin and the interior surfaces of the body such as the digestive tract, urinary tract, and lungs, as well as in sweat.

The supply of iron to the fetus increases during the last three months of pregnancy, so a full-term newborn baby has a store of about 300–500 milligrams in its body. This is an important iron store, adequate to cover the baby's needs for the first four to six months—breast milk is a poor source of the mineral, so the baby does not receive any from this source. After this, the body's iron needs increase rapidly.

Infants being introduced to solids need lots of iron. Because they have no iron stores left, their needs at this stage must be met entirely with the diet.

The need for iron increases during adolescence to support the growth spurt for both boys and girls at this time. For women, menstrual losses of iron vary from individual to individual and are mainly genetically determined. The average menstrual loss of iron has been estimated to be about 0.56 milligrams per day. This varies according to the choice of contraception used: The pill, for example, can prevent heavy blood

Daily iron needs

Iron needs vary throughout life, with females needing more than males from puberty until menopause. Thereafter, needs even out between the sexes.

AGE	IRON (MG)
0–3 months	1.7
4–6 months	4.3
7–9 months	7.8
10–12 months	7.8
1–3 years	6.9
4–6 years	6.1
7–10 years	8.7
11–18 years (boys)	11.3
11–18 years (girls)	14.8
19–50 years (males)	8.7
19–50 years (females)	14.8
50+ years (males and females)	8.7

IRON CONTENT OF FOODS

AVERAGE PORTION	IRON(mg)
One whole stewed pig's kidney (140 g)	9.0
140 g serving of stewed beef	3.8
100 g serving of sardines in tomato sauce	2.9
40 g serving of liver pâté	2.4
30 g bowl of fortified corn flakes	2.0
Six dried apricots	1.6
50 g bar of plain chocolate	1.1
One boiled egg (60g)	1.1
One medium slice of whole-grain bread	1.0
100 g serving roast chicken	0.7
One medium slice of white bread	0.6
175 g serving of boiled potatoes	0.5
20 g watercress	0.4
120 g fillet of baked cod	0.1
1 cup milk	0.1

loss, whereas an intrauterine device (IUD) usually increases menstrual blood loss.

The demand for iron increases during pregnancy. Although iron absorption does increase in response to need by up to 50 percent, women with initially low iron stores may be at increased risk of developing anemia.

Iron absorption and excretion

There are two forms of iron which are present in foods: heme and nonheme iron. Heme iron is present in meat and meat products such as red meat, liver, poultry, and fish. This form of iron makes up about 5–10 percent of the daily intake in most developed countries. Compared with nonheme iron, heme iron is absorbed relatively well—about 20–30 percent of the iron you eat is absorbed.

Nonheme iron is found in bread and grain products (made from fortified white flour), fortified breakfast cereals, green leafy vegetables, legumes, fruits, dried fruit, eggs, and dairy products. Up to 95 percent of our dietary iron is nonheme iron. Unlike heme iron, the absorption of nonheme iron is affected by the status of the body's stores. When these are depleted and when requirements are at their greatest such as in menstruating and pregnant women and growing children, absorption is increased.

Iron deficiencies

In the United States, the average adult daily intake of iron from all sources (foods and mineral supplements) is 14 milligrams for men and 12 milligrams for women. The main sources of iron are:
- cereal products—42 percent of our iron intake
- meat and meat products—23 percent
- vegetables—15 percent

Enough is enough
Growing children need iron, but it is extremely important not to exceed the RDI. Accidentally taking iron tablets is the most common cause of death from poisoning among children in the U.S.

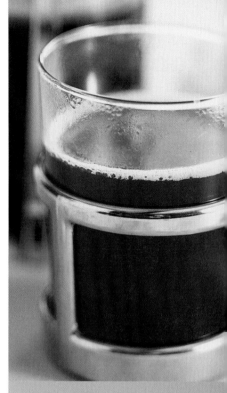

IRON STEALERS

Factors that inhibit iron absorption

Phytates and fiber-rich foods Phytates are compounds found in cereals, fiber-rich foods (particularly bran, flour, and oats), seeds, and nuts. The presence of phytates inhibits the absorption of iron and is dose related: Even a small amount of phytates have a large effect. Vitamin C in large quantities can counteract the inhibitory effects of phytates.

Tea, coffee, cocoa, spinach, and spices These contain compounds called phenols, which inhibit iron absorption.

Calcium-rich foods Foods such as milk and cheese can interfere with the absorption of iron from foods. Some studies suggest that one glass of milk reduces the absorption of iron by a half.

These intakes are within the range of the recommended daily intake (RDI) —the amount that is sufficient to meet the requirements for almost all individuals, also known as RDA— for men but below that for women.

A survey looking at the diet of young people between 4 and 18 years old found that iron intakes were low in nearly half of girls

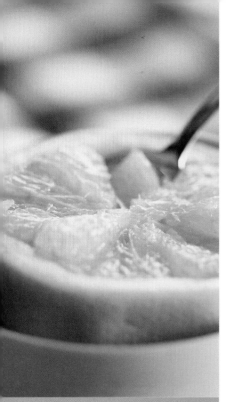

...ON-FRIENDLY FOODS

...ctors that enhance iron absorption

...tamin C-rich foods Vitamin C enhances ...e absorption of nonheme iron and is ...und in fruits, vegetables, and juices. Eating ...ood rich in vitamin C with a meal may ...uble or even triple the amount of iron ...sorbed.

...eat, fish, and seafood The presence ...these protein-rich foods in the diet ...omotes the absorption of nonheme ...n (meat also enhances the absorption ...heme iron).

...tric acid Fermented vegetables such ...sauerkraut and fermented soy sauces ...ntain citric acid, which enhances the ...sorption of nonheme iron.

between 15 and 18 years old. In this group the main sources of iron were:

- fortified breakfast cereals—about 25 percent of iron intake
- vegetables, including potatoes— 17 percent
- meat—14 percent
- bread—13 percent

Low intake of iron over a period of time can lead to iron deficiency. Iron deficiency, however, is not the same as iron deficiency anemia. In iron deficiency, the body's stores of iron are progressively reduced as a result of low levels of iron intake from the diet or from high menstrual losses. This progresses to anemia when insufficient iron is delivered to the red cells to make hemoglobin. The Centers for Disease Control uses a blood concentration of 11.9 g/dl as the standard.

Iron deficiency occurs more frequently than iron deficiency anemia. In developed countries, the prevalence of iron deficiency anemia is up to 8 percent. The rate for iron deficiency alone, however, is much higher in Western countries—the absence of iron stores is found in up to 30 percent of women of childbearing age.

Because of children's high requirements to meet tissue growth and because of menstruation in girls, young children and adolescents are particularly vulnerable to iron deficiency. Iron deficiency in preschool children and in children from some ethnic groups is common and is linked with late weaning— when solids are introduced late, because breast milk is a poor source of iron—and the early introduction of cow's milk (cow's milk is also a poor source of iron). Researchers have suggested that the lack of halal meat-based weaning foods may be responsible for low iron intakes in some children from ethnic minorities.

Excessive iron intake over a number of years can lead to health problems including liver disease and cirrhosis.

Mild iron deficiency, without anemia, is linked to reduced physical performance, mood changes, reduced ability to concentrate, and reduced resistance to infection.

Of the approximately 3.5 million people in the United States who have anemia, more than 2 million are under age 45. Anemia can be a particular problem for children and teenagers, especially girls. An estimated 9 percent of 12- to 15-year old girls are iron deficient, and 2 percent have iron deficiency anemia. About 11 percent of 18- to 19-year old girls are iron deficient and 3 percent are anemic. Teens in general are at elevated risk because they undergo rapid growth spurts. Also, because girls menstruate, they lose more iron. Many teen girls limit what they eat—particularly iron-rich foods—because they go on diets or become vegetarian. Vegetarianism is an increasingly popular lifestyle choice among all Americans, particularly teenagers. There are benefits in the reduced intake specifically of animal fat and cholesterol, but vegetarians and especially vegans—those who are still growing—have to be careful to get enough iron and protein from non-animal sources.

For elderly people, the most common cause of iron deficiency anemia is blood loss caused by undiagnosed gastrointestinal bleeding, a symptom of colon or stomach cancer.

Symptoms of iron deficiency anemia include general fatigue, lethargy, giddiness, and breathlessness on exertion.

VITAMIN B$_{12}$

Vitamin B$_{12}$ is a water-soluble vitamin that is stored in the liver. Vitamin B$_{12}$ is needed for the manufacture of nerve cells and is also required by bone marrow cells to make healthy blood.

Vitamin B$_{12}$ deficiency

In the United States, most people get enough vitamin B$_{12}$ in their daily diets. This intake is supplied by diet roughly as follows:

- Half of the vitamin B$_{12}$ we eat comes from meat and meat products.
- Milk and dairy products supply 18 percent of our B$_{12}$ intake.
- Fish and fish dishes contribute 13 percent.
- Eggs yield 8 percent.

A long-term deficiency of vitamin B$_{12}$ can cause irreversible neurological damage. Low levels of vitamin B$_{12}$ in the body can be a result of

- a poor diet;
- interaction with some types of drugs, such as some antidepressants and antibiotics and the contraceptive pill;
- interaction with alcohol;
- pernicious anemia—this prevents the absorption of vitamin B$_{12}$;
- removal of part of the intestine (commonly for Crohn's disease).

Because vitamin B$_{12}$ is contained exclusively in animal and animal products, vegetarians—particularly vegans—are at increased risk for being deficient. However, deficiency because of inadequate dietary intake is rare, because unlike other water-soluble vitamins, vitamin B$_{12}$ is stored in the liver. Isolated cases of deficiency have been reported in infants breastfed by vegan mothers and in young children on macrobiotic and vegan diets that exclude foods which have been fortified with vitamin B$_{12}$.

Low vitamin B$_{12}$ status is more common in older people and is usually caused by malabsorption in the gastrointestinal tract. A compound known as "intrinsic factor" is needed to help transport vitamin B$_{12}$ from the GI tract to the blood: In some cases, older people have lost the ability to make this factor. In other cases, deficiency is caused by a reduced ability to make the enzyme needed to release vitamin B$_{12}$ from foods. This disease tends to occur among northern Europeans, with a prevalence rate of about 10 percent after age 60.

To ensure that they do not become deficient in vitamin B$_{12}$, vegetarians and, particularly, vegans are advised to eat food, fortified with the vitamin. These include

- yeast extract;
- veggie burger mixes;
- textured vegetable protein (TVP);
- soy milks;
- vegetable and sunflower margarines; and
- breakfast cereals.

Food labels should indicate those products that have been fortified.

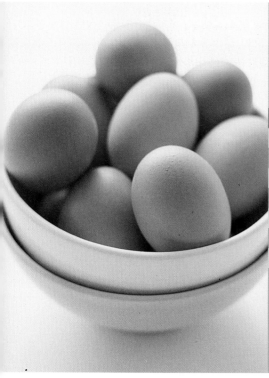

Daily B$_{12}$ needs

Vitamin B$_{12}$ is found only in animal products and in microorganisms like yeast. Liver is the richest source, but eggs, cheese, milk, meat, fish, and fortified cereals contain useful amounts.

AGE	B$_{12}$ (MCG)
0–6 months	0.3
7–12 months	0.4
1–3 years	0.5
4–6 years	0.8
7–10 years	1.0
11–18 years (boys and girls)	1.2
19–50+ years (males and females)	1.5

Breastfeeding women need an extra 0.5 mcg per day.

VITAMIN B$_{12}$ CONTENT OF FOODS

AVERAGE PORTION	B$_{12}$ (mcg)
100 g serving of fried calf's liver	58
120 g fillet of baked cod	2.4
^{4}/$_5$ cup whole milk	0.8
One boiled egg (60g)	0.66
30 g bowl of corn flakes	0.51
40 g cheddar cheese	0.44
10 g teaspoon of yeast extract	0.1

COMBATING ANEMIA

The easiest way to ensure that you do not become anemic is to make sure that your diet includes iron-rich foods and excludes those foods that limit iron absorption. For anyone who becomes anemic, there are some simple coping strategies that other sufferers found helpful while their stores were being rebuilt.

Baby boost *Use an iron-fortified formula while your baby is making the transition from milk to solid foods, and do not give babies under one year old cow's milk.*

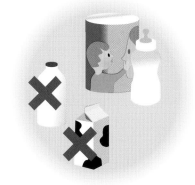

Clothes comfort *Wear loose-fitting clothes: Tight or restrictive clothing impairs your ability to breathe, which will make symptoms of anemia more acute.*

Take a seat *Sit down whenever you can—don't stand if you can sit. You could even try putting a plastic stool in the shower to sit on while showering.*

Limit tea *Limit the amount of tea you drink: Tannins—present in tea and also in red wine—interfere with iron absorption. Avoid tea with meals.*

Iron rules *Eat iron-rich foods: meat, leafy green vegetables, beans, and almonds. Remember that although liver is a rich source of iron, it should not be eaten more than once a week because it is also a concentrated source of vitamin A, which can be harmful if eaten in large amounts.*

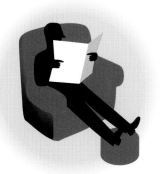

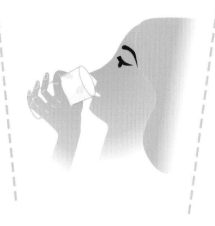

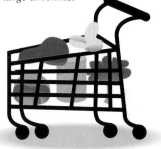

Foods for health *Increase your intake of folic acid: Many breads and cereals are fortified with this mineral, which is also present in leafy green vegetables, especially broccoli. Avoid eating calcium-rich foods at main meals but increase your intake at breakfast and as snacks.*

Fruitful combinations *Vitamin C enhances the absorption of both nonheme and heme iron, so make sure you include foods and drinks rich in this vitamin—such as fruit, vegetables, and fruit juices—with your meals.*

Slow down *Anemia saps energy. Do what you can physically: This may involve walking or moving more slowly than you are used to—but rest when you feel tired and whenever are able to, so that you conserve your energy.*

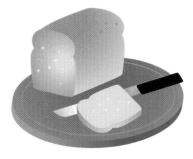

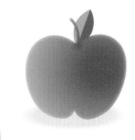

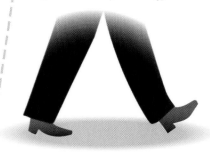

Folate and folic acid

Folate has many functions within the body: It is involved in the production of DNA (the material that carries the genetic code responsible for all our cells) and interacts with vitamin B_{12} to make healthy blood cells.

Folate is the naturally occurring form of one of the B vitamins in foods, and folic acid is the synthetic form of the vitamin used in dietary supplements or fortified foods.

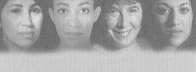

FOR WOMEN PLANNING TO CONCEIVE

There is considerable evidence to suggest that folic acid can protect against neural tube defects such as spina bifida and anencephaly if taken in the early months of pregnancy. In neural tube defects, the protective covering of the spinal cord in the fetus fails to develop properly. The protective effects of folic acid are such that the National Institutes of Health recommend that women who intend to conceive and those who are up to three months pregnant take a 400 mcg folic acid supplement each day in addition to their normal requirements from food sources. A woman who has had a pregnancy affected by a neural tube defect is advised to take a daily supplement of 5000 mcg (5 mg) in addition to the normal requirement from food (a total of 5200 mcg, or 5.2 mg).

FOLATE-RICH FOODS
Folate is present in small amounts in many different foods. Rich sources of the vitamin include
- liver;
- yeast extract;
- green leafy vegetables such as spinach, broccoli, and lettuce;
- strawberries and citrus fruits;
- legumes;
- fortified breakfast cereals; and
- fortified bread.

Most fruits, meat, milk, and dairy products contain very small amounts of folate. Because it is water soluble and heat sensitive, care must be taken when cooking foods rich in folate because at high heat it can readily be destroyed; it is also lost in large amounts of cooking water. For this reason it's best to eat fruit and vegetables raw or lightly steamed whenever possible and to choose cereals that do not require heating.

In the United States, most adults get adequate folate—400 mcg for men and women, more for pregnant and breastfeeding women—through their diet. Dietary sources are
- cereal products—21 percent of our average folate intake;

All steamed up
Folate is fragile and easily lost in too much cooking water and at high temperatures. Steaming foods rich in folate, such as vegetables, can help to preserve this important nutrient.

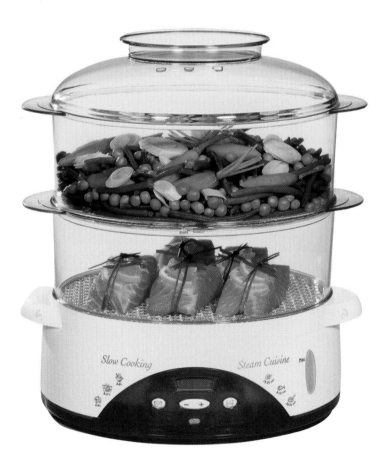

Folate

The RDI is the average dietary intake level sufficient to meet the requirements of healthy individuals at each life stage. Most diets meet recommended folate or folic acid levels.

AGE	FOLATE (MCG) RDI PER DAY
0–6 months	25
6–12 months	35
1–3 years	50
4–6 years	75
7–10 years	100
11–14 years	150
adults	400

Pregnant women require an additional 200 mcg and breastfeeding women need an extra 100 mcg per day.

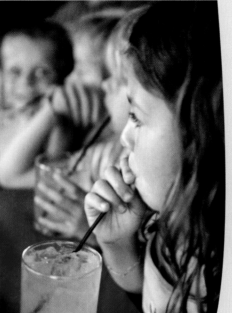

FOLATE CONTENT OF FOODS

FOOD	FOLATE (mcg) per serving
60 g black-eyed peas	126
90 g serving of steamed Brussel sprouts	99
30 g fortified breakfast cereal	75
85 g serving of steamed broccoli	54
175 g serving of boiled potatoes	46
70 g serving of steamed frozen peas	33
One medium slice of whole-grain bread	14
One medium slice of white bread	10

- vegetables—16 percent of our average folate intake;
- milk, dairy products, and meat—less than 10 percent of our average daily intake;
- fruit juices—about 5 percent of our daily intake;
- beer can be a rich source of the vitamin, providing up to 16 percent of the average intake a day in men.

THE PROBLEMS OF TOO LITTLE FOLATE

Deficiency of folate can lead to megaloblastic anemia, in which red blood cells become much larger than normal. Patients often have a sore tongue, gastrointestinal pain, anorexia, dyspepsia, constipation, or diarrhea. In addition, the nerve tissues can degenerate and there is often numbness and tingling, starting in the feet (these are similar to the symptoms of pernicious anemia).

Low levels of folate in the body can be a result of

- poor diet—folate deficiency is traditionally associated with people on low incomes and also with elderly people, who often avoid vegetables and fruit claiming that they are "difficult to eat";
- malabsorption of the vitamin in the digestive system (in celiac disease, for example);
- pregnancy, because there is an increased breakdown of folate at this time;
- interaction with some types of drugs, such as anticonvulsants; and
- interaction with alcohol, which causes decreased absorption from the digestive tract as well as increased excretion in the urine.

Recent research has shown a relationship between folate intake and the risk of cardiovascular disease. High levels of a compound called homocysteine in the blood is a risk factor for cardiovascular disease, and a moderate reduction of folate intake has been found to increase levels of homocysteine. However, trials in which diets are supplemented with folic acid to reduce homocysteine levels have not yet shown a reduction in cardiovascular disease.

Most Americans get adequate folate in their diets because since 1998, the government has required the manufacturers of certain foods—grains, cereals, and flour—to fortify them with folic acid. There is a similar proposal in England to fortify wheat flour.

Fortifying wheat flour with folic acid could reduce the number of pregnancies affected by neural tube defects by an estimated 40 percent.

Recipes for boosting iron and folate

Many foods are rich in iron or folate, so it is not difficult to get enough of these essential nutrients from the diet. The recipes here offer some delicious menu ideas.

Foods that contain iron tend to be colorful, because iron salts are pigmented— liver, red meats, and leafy green vegetables are good sources, whereas milk, for example, is not.

BEEFY POTATO SALAD

2 cloves garlic, crushed
4 tbsp tarragon
1 tbsp mustard seeds
1 tbsp fennel seeds
1 tbsp sunflower oil
1 lb beef tenderloin, trimmed of fat
1 large fennel, sliced thinly
1 lb new potatoes, halved and boiled
    until tender
1 red onion, chopped
1 large red pepper, sliced thinly
1 small red chili, seeded and sliced
juice of one lime
salt and pepper to taste
handful of chopped fresh coriander

Combine the garlic, spices, and oil, rub the mixture over the beef, and then leave it to marinate for 30 minutes. Preheat the oven to 425°F. Pan sear the beef over moderately high heat until brown on all sides, remove, and place on a preheated baking sheet and roast in the oven for 10 minutes. Reduce the heat to 375°F and roast for another 10 minutes for medium done. Remove the beef from the oven, and let it stand for 15 minutes before slicing.

Meanwhile, combine the fennel, potatoes, onion, and pepper in a serving dish, add the chili, drizzle the lime juice over the mixture, toss to mix, and adjust seasoning if necessary.

Arrange the sliced beef over the top. Sprinkle with chopped coriander just before serving.
Serves 4

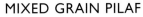

MIXED GRAIN PILAF

1½ oz quinoa

1½ oz long grain brown rice

1½ oz buckwheat

3½ cups vegetable stock

1 tbsp olive oil

1 large garlic clove, crushed

2 shallots, peeled and chopped

1 lb sieved red tomatoes

1 tbsp tomato purée

1 bay leaf

2 tbsp fresh oregano

3½ oz French green beans

3½ oz frozen peas

2 large artichoke hearts

salt and pepper to taste

juice of one lime

12 mixed green and black olives

1 lime, cut into wedges

handful flat leaf parsley, to garnish

Wash the grains. Bring the stock to a boil in a pan; add the quinoa, brown rice, and buckwheat; and cover and simmer for 30 minutes or until all the stock has been absorbed and the grains are soft.

Meanwhile, heat the oil in another pan and gently fry the garlic and shallots for 5–7 minutes or until soft. Add the tomatoes, tomato purée, and herbs and simmer for 20 minutes. Turn the heat up, add the vegetables, and cook for 5 minutes. Season and add the lime juice.

Combine the sauce and grains in a large serving bowl, and garnish with olives, lime wedges, and parsley.

Serves 4

SPINACH SALAD WITH SESAME DRESSING

1 lb young spinach leaves, washed

2 oz toasted sesame seeds

1 tsp brown sugar

2 tsp low salt soy sauce

3 tbsp dashi (fish and seaweed broth)

Blanch the spinach leaves in boiling water until they begin to wilt. Drain and set aside in a bowl. Mix the remaining ingredients together to make the dressing and pour on the spinach leaves just before serving.

Serves 4

Alcohol, blood, and the immune system

Alcohol is associated with food, socializing, and relaxation, and can be one of life's pleasures. In moderation, it may have positive health benefits, but when consumed in excess, it can have serious effects on health.

Excess alcohol dramatically increases the risk of death from liver disease, stomach cancer, pancreatitis, and car accidents.

Although less important than these problems, alcohol can also damage the immune system. Some of this damage is related to liver disease, but it can also relate to nutrition: People who drink excessively are often malnourished. Alcohol suppresses the appetite, so a drinker may not eat well. Alcohol may also inhibit the absorption of nutrients from food. Poor nutrition in turn may damage the immune system. These effects are entirely dose related: The more alcohol consumed, the more the immune system is compromised. Any quantity of alcohol that results in intoxication damages the immune system.

Alcohol also affects red blood cells. It can result in anemia, with symptoms ranging from fatigue to impaired mental capacity. It also decreases the blood's clotting ability.

ALCOHOL AND NUTRITION

In terms of nutrient content, alcohol is a source of energy, with 1 gram providing 7 calories. However, no health organization in the United States advocates the consumption of alcohol as a method of nutrient intake. However, the way in which the body processes and uses energy from alcohol is complex. Studies

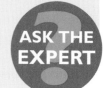

ASK THE EXPERT

ALCOHOL AND CALORIES

All alcohol contains calories. The table below shows the average calorie content of some of the most popular drinks.

ALCOHOLIC DRINK	ENERGY (KCAL)	(KJ)
1 glass of dry white wine	82	344
1 glass of sweet white wine	118	493
1 glass of red wine	85	355
1 pint of beer	184	758
1 pint of lager	167	689
1 small glass of sherry	59	245
1 single measure of hard liquor	62	257
1 measure of liqueur	64	268

have shown that when alcohol is substituted for carbohydrates, calorie for calorie, people derive less energy from alcohol than from food.

Beer does contain significant amounts of vitamin B_2 (riboflavin) and niacin, and "stouts" such as Guinness can be a good source of iron—a pint contains 1.1 milligrams. Liquor does not contain any vitamins.

Anyone who drinks to excess is running major health risks, regardless of any nutritional supplements he or she may take.

EXERCISING FOR CIRCULATORY HEALTH

Exercise plays an important part in keeping your blood and immune system healthy. Regular exercise strengthens both the heart and the leg muscles so that the blood is pumped around the body efficiently. Moderate exercise can also boost the immune system. It is never too late to start exercising, but choose appropriate activities that you will enjoy.

 76 *All forms of exercise will improve circulation by strengthening your heart and keeping your arteries and veins supple.*

 78 *A few simple lifestyle changes can help prevent or ease vein problems. Learn how diet, exercise, and even clothing can all help.*

 82 *As more people take vacations in mountainous regions, it is important to be aware of the problems high altitude can cause.*

 84 *Find out how intensive exercise can affect the immune system and what can be done to prevent overtraining.*

Exercise and circulation

Any form of exercise—vigorous or gentle—will help boost your circulation. Aerobic exercise promotes cardiovascular health, and regular stretching and flexing can relax tense and stiff muscles, enabling blood to flow freely.

CARDIOVASCULAR HEALTH

Exercise improves blood circulation by maintaining a strong heart and healthy blood vessels.

A healthy heart

The most important organ in keeping the blood flowing is the heart. The heart is a muscle, and like all muscles, it becomes stronger and more efficient with regular challenge.

At rest, the average heart pumps about 10 pints of blood per minute; during exercise, this can increase to over 42 pints per minute. The additional effort this requires strengthens and tones the heart. It is then able to pump more blood with every beat and to increase the level of pumping (if required) with less strain. This lowers the risk of heart attacks and other coronary disease.

The best type of exercise for the heart is "aerobic"—this can include jogging, skipping, bicycling, or rowing.

Artery and vein wall elasticity

Regular exercise helps keep blood vessel walls flexible. As soon as exercise begins, nerve and chemical signals stimulate the artery walls to widen in anticipation of increased blood flow. The increased movement of blood vessel walls during exercise —both expansion and contraction— ensures that they remain supple and elastic. This maintains normal blood flow and normal blood pressure. Even a simple form of exercise such as walking can improve the efficiency of blood vessels.

Blood components and pressure

Exercise also helps maintain good circulation by preventing fatty buildup in the arteries—known as atherosclerosis. This is caused by deposits of cholesterol, fats, and proteins on artery walls, which build up and form "plaque." As this plaque hardens and thickens, it significantly reduces blood flow through the artery. If blood pressure is already high, this can increase the risk of heart attack and stroke.

Regular exercise helps prevent and even reverse atherosclerosis. First, exercise lowers the amount of fat available for deposit by reducing the amount of harmful cholesterol stored in the body and carried in the blood. Second, regular exercise lowers blood pressure. This means that less cholesterol and fewer fats are forced against the artery walls. Blood pressure is further lowered when plaque on the artery walls is swept away by the increased pumping of blood during exercise.

Body temperature

During exercise, the body uses its circulatory system to regulate internal temperature. Muscles generate heat during exercise—in response, blood vessels dilate and more blood is pumped closer to the surface of the skin. As blood circulates near the surface, heat is released from the body. In the process of preventing dangerous overheating, the body keeps blood vessels healthy and improves circulation.

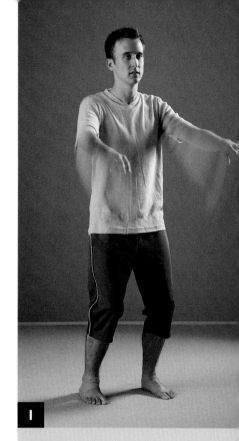

1

Exercises for boosting circulation

These exercises will warm you up and help get the blood flowing if you have become cold or stiff. Try to do exercise of this type every couple of days.

1 FULL BODY SWING Stand with both arms reaching upward. Swing both arms down past your legs as you bend your knees and curve your body forward. Then swing the arms and the body upward again. Perform several swings with real energy and you will feel the body beginning to warm up and the blood flowing.

2 POINTE WORK Contraction of the leg muscles can help the blood flow in the legs, so do these exercises regularly. Stand holding onto a wall or chair for balance. You are going to perform a 4-count movement. 1. Contract your calf muscles to raise yourself up on tiptoe. Hold this position. 2. Bend your legs (keeping your heels lifted). 3. Lower your heels slowly to the ground while

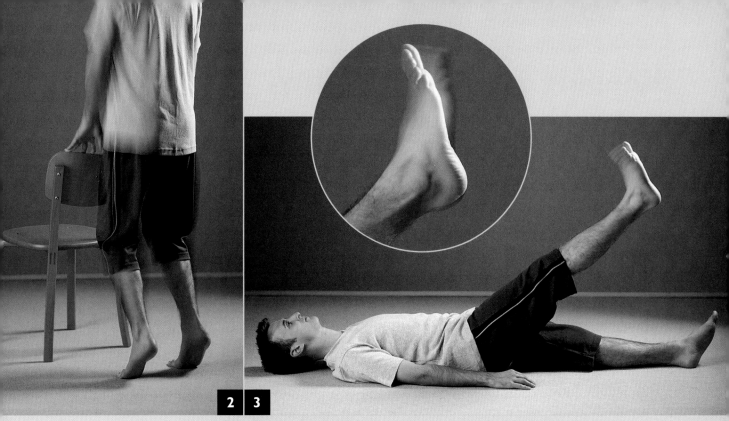

2 3

keeping your legs bent. 4. Press the legs straight. Repeat this 4-count move 10 times.

3 FLEX AND POINT Lie on the floor and lift one leg into the air. Rotate your ankle first one way and then the other. Now flex your foot (by pulling the top of the foot toward you) and then point it. Do this flex and point several times on each leg.

4 CYCLES Lie on your back and lift both legs into the air. Then revolve your legs in circles as if your were pedaling backward on a bike. This movement and the fact that your legs are lifted will aid the blood flow in the veins. Perform 10 revolutions every night.

5 AIR PRESS Lie on your back again, and this time pull your knees to your chest. Aim to keep your lower back pressed comfortably toward the floor and your hands on the floor for support. Now push both legs up into the air so that they are straight. Then push them forward at a 45-degree angle so that they are not pointed directly up toward the ceiling and they are not pushed toward the ground, which could put stress on your back. Bend them back in to the start position and repeat nine more times.

Other exercise ideas

Other good exercise options include yoga, tai chi, and walking. If you feel confident, cartwheels and handstands are great for sending blood flowing to the face and head. Massage and reflexology are also believed to improve circulation.

4 5

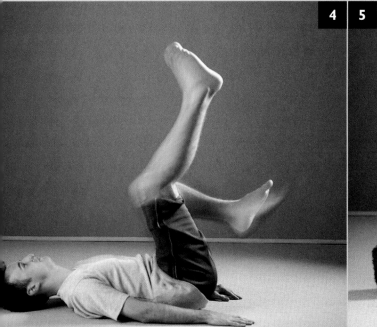

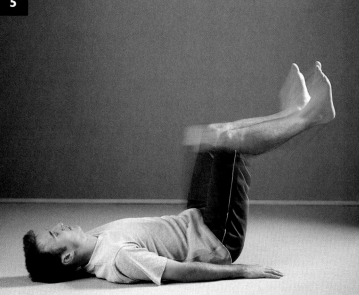

Keeping your legs healthy

Several unsightly, painful, and potentially serious circulatory conditions have their origins in the legs. Keeping your legs fit and healthy with relatively simple lifestyle changes can be beneficial, especially as you age.

VARICOSE VEINS

Varicose veins are ugly protrusions of a twisted or bulging blood vessel. These veins are usually blue in appearance and close to the surface of the skin. As they swell with blood, they can throb, feel heavy, and become uncomfortable. The legs and feet can even swell, and the skin may feel itchy. Varicose veins are most common on the back of the calves or on the inside of the legs, but they can occur in other places such as the rectum (hemorrhoids), the throat (esophageal varices), and the scrotum (varicoceles).

Causes

As blood returns to the heart after delivering oxygen around the body, the contraction of the calf and thigh muscles compresses the veins and pumps the blood upwards. The veins in the legs have one-way valves to prevent blood from flowing backward under the force of gravity. If these valves weaken and the vein walls lose their elasticity, blood collects in the veins, causing them to stretch and bulge. Circulation in the legs worsens, which can lead to painful "heavy" legs from varicose veins and other complications.

What puts you at risk?

Experts agree that the greatest determining factor as to whether someone will develop varicose veins is family history. The condition affects 10–20 percent of the population and more than 50 percent of these people have relatives who have suffered from them. Women are more affected than men, and incidence increases with age.

Lifestyle factors also play a huge part in increasing someone's risk. Obesity, for example, increases the stress placed on the veins. The extra weight presses down on the thigh and leg veins, causing them to weaken. Obesity also means extra fatty tissue, which gives less support to the veins and leads to a loss of tone in the vein walls. Age can also lead to a weakening of the supporting connective tissue.

Prolonged sitting or standing can take a toll, because they increase the pressure on the legs. This is particularly relevant for people working on their feet for long periods—people in retail, for example.

In some women, enlarged veins can first occur—or worsen—during pregnancy because of hormonal changes and the pressure caused by the growing baby.

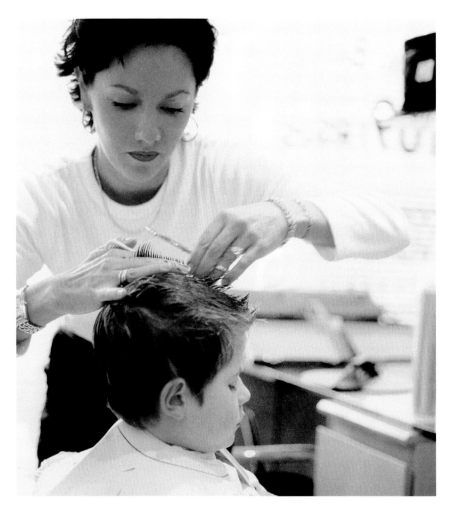

A long-standing threat
People who spend much of their working day standing in the same position, such as hairdressers, are at increased risk of developing varicose veins.

RESTLESS LEG SYNDROME

Restless leg syndrome (RLS) is a non-life-threatening but intensely irritating condition in which people suffer from an urge to move their legs. Sufferers have given this syndrome many different names, but it generally involves unusual sensations in the legs (and sometimes other parts of the body) that make the person move them in order to try to relax them.

The symptoms usually occur more in the evening, when the person is attempting to relax. Some people describe the feeling as "creepy crawlies" or "burning" up the legs, but others suffer more jerky or jumpy spasms. In many cases, it can disrupt sleep patterns and has been known to cause injury to the person's sleeping partner.

It is not known what causes the condition, although in some cases it may be nerve damage. It is not even known, at this time, where the RLS impulses are generated, although there is some new evidence that points to a linkage of chromosomes 5 and 10. There is also a genetic link, so the condition tends to run in families. The most common sufferers of RLS include middle aged people (the condition gets worse with age), women who are pregnant, and individuals under stress. People with poor circulation or anemia may also suffer.

What can you do to relieve the symptoms of RLS?

- Iron or folic acid supplements can be given to protect against anemia.
- Good hydration and relaxation techniques may help with stress and tiredness.
- Restricted caffeine intake is recommended. Although caffeine was believed to reduce symptoms, it really only delays their intensity.
- A balanced diet (with plenty of fruit, vegetables, and carbohydrates; modest amounts of protein and dairy products; and a limited amount of fat and sugar) will help keep the body's systems healthy.

Bedtime routine

These gentle stretches may help.

1 Lie on your back on the bed and lift one leg straight up toward the ceiling so that you can feel a stretch in the back of your leg. Then bend the leg in toward you and hold it with both hands. Release and extend the leg back to the ceiling. Repeat with the other leg.

2 Raise one leg and gently circle the whole leg, drawing a circle on the ceiling with your foot. Move the leg in a circular motion, slowly mobilizing the joint at the hip and thigh. Circle the leg eight times in one direction and then in the other. Repeat with the other leg.

3 Finally, raise both legs as straight as you can and push your heels toward the ceiling. You will feel a stretch in the back of the legs—the hamstring muscles.

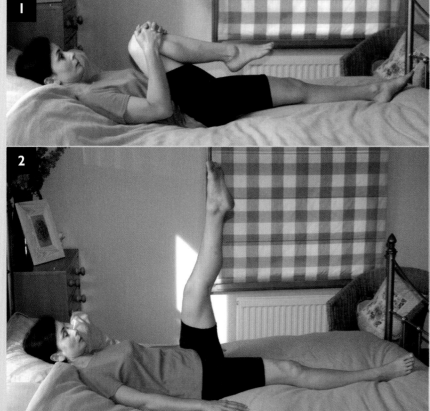

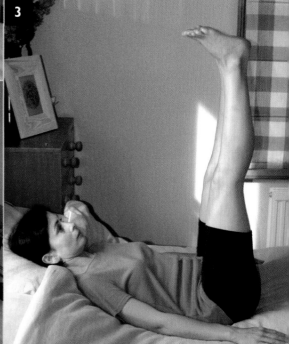

Preventing varicose veins

The best way to avoid varicose veins is to follow guidelines for staying healthy. Keep your weight within the recommended range for your height, and exercise regularly. Exercising will provide regular contractions of the muscles, thereby helping blood flow and circulation.

Try to avoid standing or sitting for long periods of time, but if you have to, be sure to regularly lift your heels and flex your feet to contract the calves. Try to take regular breaks during which you walk around to keep the blood flowing. Do not cross your legs when sitting and watch your posture—sit upright so you do not pressurize certain areas. Practice lifting your legs when lying down and performing some backward cycling movements with the legs.

As a general rule, your diet should be low in fat and high in fiber. Some experts suggest a diet rich in bioflavonoids (found in dark green leafy vegetables), and extra vitamin C and E may help. You should drink plenty of fluids (particularly water) so you do not become dehydrated. You should also restrict your intake of caffeine and alcohol.

If you suspect you may be susceptible to varicose veins, opt for loose-fitting garments and wear support tights in addition to following the above guidelines.

There is no definitive prevention or even cure. The disorder is progressive and although sclerotherapy (which seals off small varicose veins) or stripping of larger veins gets rid of the immediate problem, the procedure merely diverts the burden of blood flow to other veins which can, in turn, become varicose.

DEEP VENOUS THROMBOSIS (DVT)

A thrombosis is a blood clot in a deep vein. Superficial and deep veins run throughout the body, and if a blood clot forms in the valve of a deep vein, it can block the whole vein and stop blood flow, causing painful cramps. There is potentially fatal danger if a part of the blood clot breaks away from the main one (the embolus) and travels. If the whole clot travels further in the bloodstream, it can block a blood vessel in the lungs or brain or even in the placenta of a growing baby.

DVT was first noticed during World War II, among people sitting still for hours in air-raid shelters.

What causes DVT?

One of the major risk factors for deep vein thrombosis is staying still for too long. Blood clots can form during a period of just a few hours if the legs are not exercised.

DVT is often called "economy class syndrome" because a higher frequency of the problem was noticed in travelers sitting in cramped seats. DVT is not restricted to economy class fliers, however, or even to long-haul flights. It can affect sales reps, truck drivers, or people who sit for long periods at a desk.

The sitting position can restrict circulation around the legs. The less active the muscles in the leg are, the fewer signals they send to the brain to send sufficient blood to them. The blood that does get to the legs may not circulate as efficiently as normal, and clots can develop.

Who is at risk?

People are at higher risk of developing DVT if they
- are over the age of 40;
- have had blood clots already;
- have a family history of blood clots;
- have cancer or have had treatment for cancer in the past;
- are being treated for heart disease; or
- have had recent surgery, particularly on the hips or knees.

DVT is also more common in women who
- are pregnant;
- have recently had a baby;
- are taking the contraceptive pill; or
- are on hormone replacement therapy.

Does aspirin reduce the risk of developing DVT?

There is currently no direct evidence that aspirin reduces the risk of travel-related DVT. It is known, however, to make the platelets (part of the blood clotting mechanism) less "sticky." If your doctor agrees, take one aspirin a day for three days before your trip. If you are already taking aspirin, do not increase your dose. Aspirin should not be seen as a "quick fix" solution. In a recent study of 1,000 airline passengers, some of those who took aspirin still developed blood clots. It appears that aspirin may give a false sense of security, encouraging people to sleep throughout the flight, thereby increasing the risk of DVT.

ASK THE EXPERT

Between 90 and 95 percent of all people who develop DVT are in one or more of these groups.

People who are overweight, elderly, have to stand in one place for a long time, or have to endure long periods of bed rest may also be at risk. Certain trauma situations and medications can also trigger DVT.

What are the symptoms?

Symptoms may include redness, swelling, and heat in the area. There may also be pain, discoloration, or ulceration over the area where the vein lies, or joint pain and soreness. Other symptoms may include fever, a rapid heartbeat, or a sudden unexplained cough. Sometimes there are no symptoms at all if the thrombus occurs in a vein that is not in the arm or leg.

Treatment

DVT is treated with blood-thinning drugs or anticoagulants. These work by interfering with the body's natural coagulation process, preventing blood from thickening into the semi-solid state that precedes clotting.

Contrary to popular belief, blood thinners don't dissolve clots—the body does. This natural process is called fibrinolysis. Anticoagulants can keep clots from enlarging, however, which is critical. The three types of anticoagulants used to treat DVT are unfractionated heparin (UFH), low molecular weight heparins (LMWH), and coumadin, which is a long-term treatment.

Reducing your risk

An active lifestyle—which includes regular exercise—will keep your body well-conditioned. This is a major factor in preventing DVT.

PREVENTATIVE MEASURES FOR TRAVELERS

Keeping your blood flowing while sitting for long periods is the important issue. Experts recommend the following when traveling for long periods:

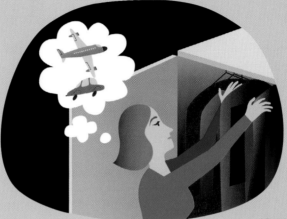

When traveling, make sure you dress in comfortable nonrestrictive clothing. Wear comfortable slip-on shoes if possible.

Drink plenty of water before and during the journey to keep well hydrated. Avoid caffeine, alcohol, and smoking.

Support stockings, worn during a trip, have been shown to reduce the risk of DVT.

When on a plane, get up and walk around every hour. If you can, try to get an aisle seat for extra room to move your legs. If you are a passenger in a car, try propping your feet up on the dashboard or seat in front of you and flexing and extending your feet. If you are the driver, when stationary, work your thigh muscles by lifting your knees up to touch the steering wheel. Then press your feet hard against the floor.

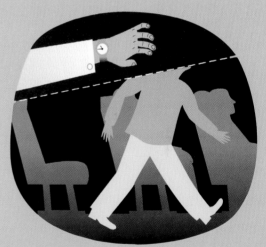

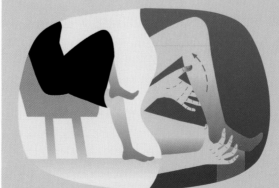

When it is impossible to walk around—if you are required to keep your seat belt on, for instance—place one foot on the other knee and knead and massage the foot and calf using upward motions of the hand to help circulation. Don't cross your legs at the knee.

Exercise and altitude

High altitude exercise can be great fun, but it can also have serious effects for anyone who is unprepared. A few precautionary measures can ensure the enjoyment of high altitude activities such as climbing, skiing, biking, or hiking.

The effects of altitude on exercise were first investigated following the 1968 Olympic Games in Mexico City. Here, where the elevation is 7500 feet, for the first time ever there were no world records achieved in events lasting longer than two and a half minutes. The Africans, however, who regularly trained at high altitude, dominated the endurance events.

Now, with more understanding of the effects of altitude on the body's systems, many competing athletes—at all levels—are building altitude adjustments into their pre-competition training.

It's not just athletes who experience the effects of exercising at high altitude. Increasing numbers of people enjoy skiing, hiking, and activity vacations in high altitude regions every year. Unfortunately, many people are not aware of how the change in altitude will affect them and do not allow for a period of adjustment. By rushing into activities too quickly, they lose valuable days of their vacation to fatigue or illness.

EXERCISING AT ALTITUDE

The main effect on the body of exercising at high altitudes is a reduction in cardiovascular capacity: Higher than 5000 feet, there is a 10–11 percent reduction for each 3000 foot ascent. This means that at an altitude of 6500–8000 feet, an individual will only be able to perform at 90 percent of his or her sea level capacity.

High levels of muscle fatigue are also common because each lungful of air contains less oxygen, and this oxygen is consumed during exercise.

Such physiological challenges are not serious, and cardiovascular capacity will improve with regular high altitude exercise. It is important, however, for individuals to understand their limitations and to decrease their workload, resistance, and pace, particularly upon arrival.

THE BODY'S RESPONSE

At high altitude, the air is "thinner." This doesn't mean that there is less oxygen (this remains stable at 20.9 percent) but that there is less pressure.

With each breath, less oxygen is taken, via the lungs, into the bloodstream and around the body—resulting in a diminished oxygen supply to the muscles and other tissues. This is known as hypoxia.

Hypoxia has wide-ranging symptoms, although most of these are considered to be normal adjustments to altitude conditions. One of the earliest symptoms is impairment of judgement—similar to mild intoxication. This can initially be felt as a mild headache or slight disorientation. Shortness of breath is another indication of low oxygen levels. The body responds by increasing the ventilation rate (rapid breathing) and cardiac output (faster heart rate) to raise the amount of oxygen available for tissues. These symptoms usually disappear over 24–48 hours.

ACUTE MOUNTAIN SICKNESS

More serious symptoms of hypoxia indicate the onset of acute mountain sickness (AMS). These include worsening headache, nausea, fatigue, dizziness, acute tunnel vision, slurred speech, staggering walk, memory loss, or a combination of these.

AMS is a frequent problem for climbers, and it commonly occurs above 10,000 feet. It is caused by ascending too high too quickly. The key to managing AMS is to ascend slowly because acclimatization takes time. Above 10,000 feet, the daily ascent rate should be no greater than 1000 feet per day. Increasingly, however, factors such as limited vacation time, the increase in the number of high-altitude roads, and rapid ascent in cable cars can lead to this basic rule being ignored.

Mild AMS can be treated with rest and a halt in the ascent, plus aspirin or acetaminophen to relieve the headache. The symptoms should disappear within 48 hours. Severe AMS should be treated with descent, oxygen, and Diamox (the standard drug for altitude sickness, which stimulates an increase in breathing).

ACCLIMATIZATION

The body adjusts to high altitude by making more red blood cells to enable more oxygen to be carried in the bloodstream. When the kidneys intially detect the lower level of oxygen in the blood, they release a hormone called erythropoietin. This triggers the bone marrow to start producing more red blood cells within 24–48 hours.

To make room for the increasing number of red blood cells, the body gets rid of fluid from the blood— urine output increases, and fluid can collect in the body's tissues. The increase in proportion of red blood cells compared to the plasma (liquid portion) of the blood is called hemoconcentration or "thick blood." Initially the body gets rid of 10–15 percent of the blood's plasma. Full acclimatization over two weeks would increase a person's red blood cell count by 30–50 percent.

HIGH ALTITUDE ADVICE

One of the main problems to be aware of at altitude, particularly when exercising, is dehydration. This can be caused by increased breathing and the relatively low humidity of mountainous areas and airplane cabins. Sweating while exercising also causes dehydration—as the body cools itself by sweating, 2–4 pints of fluid can be lost per hour. In addition, the increased urinary output caused by the process of hemoconcentration leads to dehydration. This means that the blood becomes thicker and that blood flow can become more sluggish. Without hydration, unconditioned people are at risk of thrombosis.

It is vital to keep well hydrated. Drink regularly during and after exercise, and replace lost fluids with water. Caffeine and alcohol should be avoided if possible because they are diuretics. Avoid salty foods and overeating: These can magnify the effects of high altitude. Ask for a humidifier in your room to increase the water content in the air and relieve dried out sinuses.

Protection from altitude exposure
Ensure that you wear clothing designed for altitude conditions. High-SPF sunscreen is also recommended because ultra-violet radiation increases by 5 percent for every 1000 feet of altitude.

Getting the balance right

It seems odd, but athletes catch more colds than people in sedentary occupations. Why is this? To understand, we need to look in detail at the effects exercise can have on the immune system.

Studies have shown that many high-performance athletes can have chronically weakened immune systems. Indeed, it could be said that in immunological terms, at particular points in their training and competition schedules, elite athletes are extremely unhealthy. Many athletes report significant bouts of upper respiratory tract infection (URTI), which include the common cold, acute sore throat, laryngitis, bronchitis, ear infection, and the flu.

During both the winter and summer Olympic Games, clinicians report that URTIs are the most frequent and irksome health problems athletes experience— they affect performance and can jeopardize years of training.

It appears that the main factor that determines the condition of the immune system is the intensity and duration of the exercise.

MODERATE EXERCISE BOOSTS IMMUNITY

Regular moderate exercise has been shown to stimulate immune function. Positive immune changes take place during each bout of moderate activity. The numbers and activity of natural killer cells increase, and T cell function improves. There is also increased blood flow and movement of blood cells.

Although the immune system returns to preexercise levels very quickly after the exercise session is over, each session represents a boost

that translates into fewer days of sickness and appears to reduce the risk of infection over the long term. Studies show that 60–90 percent of people who exercise regularly experience fewer URTIs than those who don't exercise.

IMMUNOSUPPRESSION

Although regular moderate exercise leads to fewer URTIs, evidence suggests that intense training and competition actually suppress some aspects of the immune response.

Intensive exercise initially causes a stimulation of the immune system, but for 3–72 hours after exercise, there is a general impairment of the immune system that leaves athletes vulnerable to infection.

Stress response

The body perceives high-intensity exercise as stressful and responds by releasing the stress hormones epinephrine and cortisol into the bloodstream. It appears that it is the fluctuating levels of these hormones which cause many of the immune system changes.

During intense exercise there is a rise in granulocytes (monocytes and neutrophils) and lymphocytes. Among the lymphocytes—which include T cells, B cells and natural killer (NK) cells—NK cells increase the most during exercise. However, these levels fall within five minutes of the exercise ending, and within 30–60 minutes, there is a dramatic

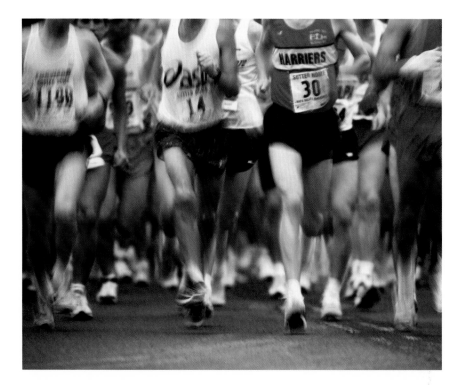

Energy needs on the run
Athletes should think about their energy needs on an hour-by-hour basis, not just from day to day. Drinking carbohydrate sports drinks during a long-distance race can help maintain steady blood sugar levels.

reduction in both the number and activity of lymphocytes. NK cells in particular, plummet to levels 25–30 percent lower than preexercise— a direct result of the cortisol released into the bloodstream. NK activity remains low for 3–6 hours after intense exercise. In addition, the cortisol released during intense exercise causes a decrease in the plasma levels of glutamine, which T cell lymphocytes depend on for optimal growth, so their function is diminished. Intense exercise also causes an increase in free radicals, which cause damage to immune cells.

"Open window"

The cumulative effect of these immunological changes results in a less effective defense system. This is why scientists speak of an "open window" theory, which highlights a postexercise period in which athletes are vulnerable. In the 3–72 hours that immunity is lowered, bacteria and viruses gain a foothold, increasing the risk of infection, especially URTIs.

Alberto Salazar caught 12 colds in 12 months of training before winning gold in the 1984 Olympic marathon.

One of the largest studies to date was carried out in 1987, when 2311 participants in the Los Angeles marathon were followed for two months before and one month after the race. Runners who actually ran were compared with those who had signed up but did not run for reasons other than illness. The researchers found that one in seven runners

---

10–18 YEARS

Overtraining and teenagers

It is especially important for children and adolescents to avoid the risks of high-intensity training.

- **Overuse injuries** Excessive stress or overload can lead to tissue breakdown and injury. Typical overuse injuries are repetitive stress injuries, injuries to developing joint surfaces, and injuries to the developing spine.
- **Sexual maturation** Athletic girls tend to experience their first period later or find that their periods stop (amenorrhea) because of training stress and low levels of body fat. Training has no adverse effect on male maturation.

- **Nutrition** A healthy diet is critical for young athletes. An iron deficiency can lead to "sports anemia," and a calcium deficiency can lead to increased bone fractures. Eating disorders are a risk for female athletes, particularly in sports in which low body weight is deemed "ideal."

To train without overtraining,
- Avoid excessive training.
- Take scheduled rest periods.
- Include conditioning and flexibility.
- Experiment with different sports.
- Watch for warning signs of overtraining and "burnout."

---

developed a cold in the week after the marathon, which was six times the nonrunner rate.

OVERTRAINING

Exercising every day for an hour or more at 85 percent of your maximum heart rate can be considered overtraining. This can lead to a range of symptoms including recurrent URTIs, general fatigue, slow recovery, irritability, depression, poor concentration, and sleep disturbance.

To check if you are overtraining, you can try the Rusko test. Lie quietly for 10 minutes at the same time every day and monitor your heart rate—this should stay constant for each 10-minute period. Stand up and check your heart rate exactly 15 seconds after standing, and then obtain your average heart rate during

the period 90–120 seconds after standing. If you are on the verge of overtraining, your standing rate will increase over a period of a few weeks. Knowing this will give you a chance to ease back on training.

SENSIBLE GUIDELINES

- Ensure that you get plenty of rest to enable your body to adapt to intense training.
- Try to avoid contact with people who have colds.
- Warm up well and keep warm during competitions.
- Take vitamin supplements (vitamin C and zinc) for cold symptoms.
- If you have a cold, reduce training for 1–2 weeks. If you have the flu or bronchitis, stop training for 3–4 weeks to prevent damage to your heart—this can be life-threatening.

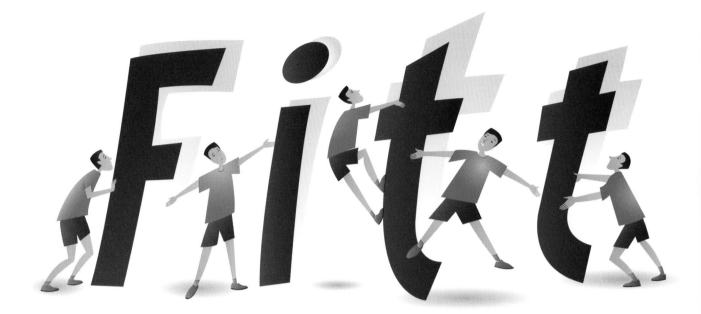

Frequency:

Whether your goal is to control weight or to get in shape, the frequency should be 3–5 times a week.

Intensity:

Exercise should make you feel energized, not exhausted. Increase intensity slowly—start by walking longer or faster.

Time:

Try about 30 minutes of exercise at each session. Daily activities such as walking, gardening, and climbing stairs all count.

Type:

The more types of exercise you get, the better. Moderate exercise involving rhythmic leg movements is best.

THE FITT PRINCIPLE

It is not just a question of how often and how long you exercise but also how hard and what type—called the FITT principle: Frequency, Intensity, Time, and Type.

Frequency

Experts say that cardiovascular exercise should be done at a frequency of 3–5 days a week. This may seem difficult, but it doesn't mean you have to go to the gym each time. It can include daily activities such as gardening, walking, cleaning, and climbing stairs. Obviously, attending appropriate fitness classes helps too. Beginners should start with three days a week, skipping a day between sessions.

Intensity

Start with an endurance-based activity like walking and gradually build up to more vigorous exercise. Increase the intensity slowly and never exercise to exhaustion. You can measure the intensity at which you are exercising in a number of ways:

- Your cardiovascular level may be gaged by your ability to hold a conversation while exercising.
- Check your heart rate at intervals: It should be no more than 80 percent of your maximum heart rate (220 minus your age).
- Use self-perception to gage how hard you are working on a scale of 1–16, where 1 is easy and 16 is extremely hard.

Time

The duration of the aerobic portion of an exercise session should be between 12 and 60 minutes. The less fit you are, the shorter the duration and the more frequently you should exercise. As you become fitter, you can exercise less often for longer periods.

Type

A useful approach is to try as many different types of activity as possible. Your body will be less likely to become accustomed to any one type. Trying different exercises also lessens the chances of overuse of any one body part. You are also less likely to get bored.

The positive effects of exercise

Regular exercise is good for you. It makes you stronger and it gives you better endurance and more energy. It also provides you with increased self-confidence and enhances concentration.

Exercise promotes an increase in "good" cholesterol and lowers blood pressure, thereby decreasing the risk of heart attack and stroke. Regular exercise makes you more relaxed and this can boost your immune system. It also has been credited with lowering rates of certain cancers.

PROTECTING YOURSELF

The immune system is under daily threat from infections. In addition to building the system up through lifestyle factors such as diet, there are two major ways in which you can support it: vaccination against many diseases and avoiding behaviors that might compromise the system.

 88 *Since the first vaccination was carried out more than 200 years ago, the process has become a first line of defense against disease.*

 92 *Understanding the risks of infection is an important first step in helping the immune system work effectively.*

Why vaccination matters

The process of vaccination is one of the greatest success stories of modern medicine, offering the best defense against an expanding range of deadly diseases by giving treatments months, even years, before they are likely to be contracted.

Smallpox vaccination has brought about the complete eradication of the disease's deadly microbes from the environment. The World Health Organization (WHO) is currently targeting other diseases—including polio—for similar treatment in the hope that they will be eliminated as a result. Despite such global success, as well as regional population-based

Raising healthy kids
The infant death rate has fallen steadily in the last 50 years in the U.S., to its current rate of 7 in 1000. Vaccination has played a major part in this success.

improvements—for example, the virtual eradication of infections due to Haemophilus influenzae type b meningitis in those countries that are now using the Hib vaccine—safety concerns have prompted many people to question the value of immunization.

THE DANGER OF SKEPTICISM
The process of immunization involves taking a treatment long before a disease is contracted, often in the knowledge that an individual's risk of contracting the disease is low. As such, the process requires a

strong belief that it will generally do more good than harm. It is important that up-to-date information is available on the balance of risks and benefits because circumstances can change every year.

A single dose of the MMR vaccine for measles, mumps, and rubella will offer approximately 90 percent of vaccinated children complete protection against measles. However, if only 92 percent of children—rather than 100 percent—receive the vaccine, only 83 percent of all children are protected. U.S. schools usually report about 95 percent immunization.

Despite a good vaccine and impressive uptake, therefore, many children remain unprotected, allowing epidemics to develop. If the number of vaccinated children

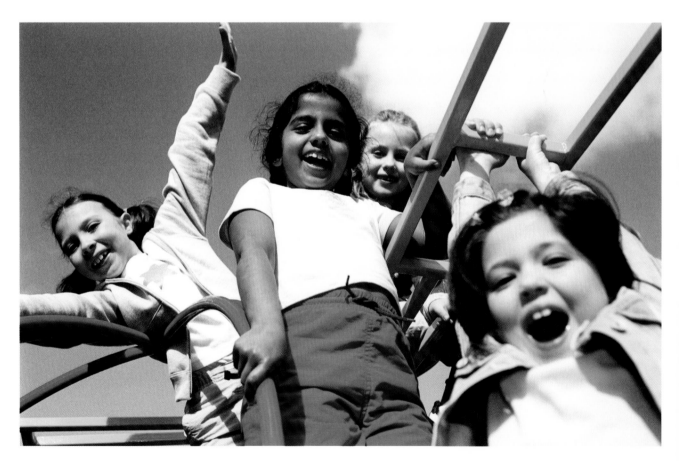

falls further, the situation becomes worse, changing the overall risk-to-benefit ratio and increasing the need for immunization.

Because these infections have become rare, many of us have forgotten how dangerous they are; measles is a killer, mumps can cause sterility, and rubella causes birth defects.

At the other end of the scale is polio, which has been largely removed from some parts of the world, including the Americas and Europe, through vaccination. As a result, even though the risk of giving a child the vaccine is very low, the risk of contracting the disease may be even lower in these areas.

Custom vaccination

We know that vaccinations are very low risk because such treatments are among the most commonly administered in the world, and they give us more data about their effects than almost any other type of treatment. However, a "one injection fits all" policy will inevitably not fit all or, therefore, protect all. Developments in the science of human genetics may lead to a more personalized process. In the future, genetic testing may indicate which people are more likely to suffer from a particular adverse reaction and who will require more booster inoculations in order to be protected. In addition to this, new vaccines are constantly being developed, and this may make immunization more important as the number of diseases they are able to combat increases.

IMMUNIZING CHILDREN

During the first six months of life, we are usually protected from many common diseases by antibodies that

In 1967, when the WHO launched its eradication initiative, smallpox affected 15 million people annually; by 1980 the disease had been eliminated worldwide.

have been passed on to us from our mothers. This gives babies a brief period of time to build up strength before they face the serious challenge of infectious disease, which in some parts of the world kills as many as one in six children under five. Fortunately, this six-month period can now be used to immunize children so that as their mother's antibodies become less potent, they get additional help in combating infections when they meet them, greatly increasing their chance of surviving their first year.

Currently, immunizations that are available for use during this period protect against diphtheria, tetanus, whooping cough (pertussis) —all in one vaccine called DTP— polio, meningitis group C, and haemophilus. In addition, immunizations against tuberculosis (TB), hepatitis B, chicken pox (varicella), and meningitis group A may be given if the risks are thought to be high enough. "High risk" is usually defined as

- close contact with somebody known to be suffering from active disease (usually the mother in the case of varicella) or
- living in (or visiting) a country—or a city or area—where there is a high prevalence of the specific disease.

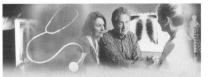

Milestones
IN MEDICINE

Edward Jenner had been an English country doctor for 24 years when he first tested his ideas on immunization. At the time, smallpox was the biggest killer, with 10 percent of the UK population dying from it each year. In 1796, intrigued by stories that people who caught cowpox from their herds did not contract smallpox— even if several other family members caught the disease— Jenner took the pus from a milkmaid with cowpox and put it into cuts made into an eight-year-old boy's arm. The boy suffered what appeared to be a normal, mild, cowpox infection. A few weeks later, Jenner risked being accused of murder and repeated the experiment using smallpox pus. The boy remained healthy, and the concept of immunization was born.

It is possible to protect against mumps, measles, and rubella using the MMR vaccine when a baby is 12 months old.

For those at high risk, the pneumococcal vaccine can be given to children over two years old and the typhoid vaccine after age six. Vaccination against yellow fever is also possible.

Adult immunization programs are essentially the same as those for children, and most adults can be inoculated to "catch up" at virtually any age.

Does homeopathic immunization work?

Scary stories in the media regarding the potential side effects and occasional ineffectiveness of traditional vaccinations have led to a rise in interest in homeopathic alternatives to immunization. Although such alternatives exist, they are not considered acceptable substitutes for state-mandated vaccinations. Whether the homeopathic remedies work or not or have any side effects is not known because no real scientific studies have been undertaken.

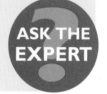

ASK THE EXPERT

TRAVELING THE WORLD

Guidelines for vaccines required for traveling vary depending on where you are going, so a clear plan of destinations is essential. Your doctor will have a list. You can also check the Centers for Disease Control Web site. Typical vaccine options are meningococcal ACWY or AC, Japanese encephalitis, rabies, tickborne encephalitis, typhoid, hepatitis A and B, and yellow fever. Yellow fever is now the only disease for which an international vaccination certificate may be required for entry into a country following travel from a country where it is endemic. This also used to be the case with cholera, but the legislation has now been dropped because the World Health Organization (WHO) has accepted that the vaccine was not effective at preventing transfer of the infection from one country to another. This vaccine is no longer recommended for any traveler.

In theory, each individual travel vaccine should be given its own 10-day period to take effect. In practice, however, because of time constraints, many vaccines can be given at the same time without apparent adverse effects. Courses of most travel vaccines, plus any single dose vaccines, can be administered over a four-week period. Final doses should be completed before the departure date to allow immunity to develop. It can take up to four weeks, for example, for full immunity to develop following a Japanese encephalitis vaccination, and it should be given at least two weeks before departure in case a delayed allergic reaction occurs. Your doctor or a travel clinic can offer good advice on an immunization schedule.

If children are traveling, they can be given many vaccines earlier than the standard schedule (and often from birth). It must be remembered, however, that if this is done, they may require additional boosters later in life because the immunity from early immunization does not seem to be as long-lasting.

On returning from the tropics it is advisable to visit your doctor, even if you are feeling well. It may be that a disease can be detected (for example in a stool sample) before symptoms develop, allowing for more effective treatment.

Mosquitoes can bite through thin material, so spray clothes with an insecticide such as permethrin (which may last up to two weeks).

In the evenings, wear long-sleeved shirts and long pants, protect exposed skin with a repellent containing diethyltoluamide (DEET), and wear DEET-soaked ankle and wristbands. DEET preparations are usually only effective for two hours, so frequent application is required. Be careful when applying it to the face: It can irritate mucus membranes (do a skin test first).

When a bedroom cannot be made safe from insects, use a permethrin-impregnated bed net (which is much more effective than an ordinary net).

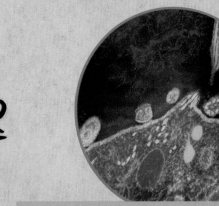

For diseases for which there is no effective vaccine, such as malaria and HIV/AIDS, a more involved protection program is required. In the case of malaria, this means visiting your doctor before and after travel, taking the right antimalaria tablets, and protecting yourself from mosquito bites. Protection against HIV includes behavior changes—using barrier contraceptives and perhaps chemical prophylactics.

Sleep in air-conditioned or screened accommodations. Rooms should be sprayed with an insecticide every evening after sundown to eliminate mosquitoes that may have entered during the day.

Avoiding risky behavior

One of the biggest threats to the immune system is HIV, which can—but does not necessarily—slowly break it down. There is a lot a person can do to reduce the risk of getting HIV or of passing it on, and to stay healthy even after a diagnosis.

HIV is the human immunodeficiency virus. The virus can, but does not always, lead to AIDS—acquired immune deficiency syndrome. AIDS is not a single disease but a collection of the most common illnesses that characteristically affect people living with HIV.

There are approximately 850,000–950,000 people in the United States infected with HIV; many—25 percent—are unaware of the infection. There has been a lot of misunderstanding about HIV transmission, as well as misinformation about who is at risk and who isn't.

HIV is passed on in three main ways:
• Through unprotected penetrative sex (anal or vaginal) between someone who is HIV positive and someone who is HIV negative.
• By getting HIV-infected blood into the bloodstream: This can happen when someone who is HIV positive and someone who is HIV negative share needles when injecting drugs. It does not happen through blood transfusions anymore.
• A woman can pass the virus to her baby during childbirth.

HIV does not discriminate on the grounds of age, sex, gender, class, race, or sexuality. It is an individual's behavior—and the behavior of his or her partner—that puts that individual at risk.

For transmission to take place sexually, there must be a partner who has the virus and a partner who does not and a route of transmission out of one body and into the other. HIV doesn't emerge as a result of having sex, so unprotected sex between two people who do not have the virus cannot magically produce it, as some people think.

Many people are unaware of the dangers of risky behavior, and this ignorance is directly affecting the rate at which HIV is spreading, particularly among heterosexual people in the United States.

TRANSMISSION AND ORAL SEX

There have been a handful of cases of transmission through oral sex worldwide, but these should be put within the context of how much oral sex is going on. It seems that some very specific conditions have to be in place for oral sex to be a transmission route for infection. Bleeding gums, cuts, or sores in the mouth and inflammation caused by common throat infections, allergies, or sexually transmitted infections such as gonorrhoea, are likely to aid transmission. Again, there must be a route of transmission of the virus from a partner with HIV to a partner without HIV. It seems that vaginal and anal sex are more likely transmission routes.

OTHER RISKY BEHAVIOR

Injecting intravenous drugs is a bad idea for many reasons, but it is vital that users do not share needles. The risk of HIV and hepatitis being

HIV AND TATTOOS

HIV is actually a delicate virus which cannot survive long outside the human body. It is usually only transmitted when enough infected blood is introduced into a body. The structure of tattoo needles makes HIV transmission by this route unlikely. It seems that there has never been a case of transmission in this way in the United States, and in cases reported elsewhere, the affected individuals were deemed "high risk" for contracting the virus whether they got a tattoo or not.

The main risk when getting a tattoo is infection with hepatitis, a hardy virus that can survive for long periods outside the human body and can be transmitted by an infected needle. Reputable tattooists
• sterilize all equipment thoroughly;
• use new needles for each client;
• use individual portions of ink and lubricant;
• dispose of used needles following health department guidelines; and
• clean chairs between clients.

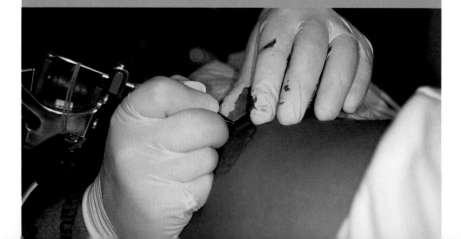

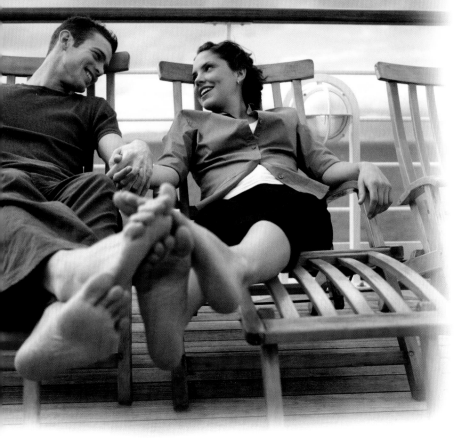

transmitted in this way is high. In some areas, needle exchange programs have been introduced with the goals of ensuring that users have access to sterile needles, that they have access to medical staff, and that there is also social and psychological support available if they want to stop taking the drugs. Where such programs have been set up, studies indicate that HIV infection rates appear to be falling.

THE BODY AND HIV

HIV works differently from a lot of other infections. It doesn't just try to get into the body and do some damage, it actually finds and attacks the CD4 cells (helper T cells) that are the "organizers" of the immune system. When HIV moves into an individual's CD4 cells and kills some of them off, the immune system stops working as well as it should. When HIV first gets into the body, a person may get a sore throat, fever, or rash, although the vast majority of patients have no symptoms when

HIV prevention

Of the 40,000 new infections in the United States per year, 15 percent of men and 85 percent of women are infected through heterosexual sex. Half of these new cases occur in people under 25.

they are first infected. Although HIV attacks the immune system, the body does make antibodies against the virus. These antibodies are present from a few weeks after infection first takes place. The HIV test consists of checking the presence of these antibodies and is nearly 100 percent reliable.

Having a test

There is one very good reason to have a test if you suspect that you may have been infected: If you know you have HIV, you can do something about it. There is no cure for HIV and there is still a lot of prejudice attached to those people living with the virus, so having a test is a difficult decision for many people to make. On the other hand, it can

prevent unnecessary worrying, and many people find that once they know for sure, they have some relief. Before you have a test, you should be offered pretest counseling to make sure you completely understand the consequences of testing. You must be asked permission for the test to be done: It can never be done without your consent. There is enormous support from charities offering counseling and basic information on social issues as well as on legal and financial matters (see page 160).

IT'S NOT TRUE!

The myths surrounding HIV

Contrary to popular belief, HIV is a fragile virus that is not easily passed on. Here are three common myths on HIV infection.

"You can get HIV from a mosquito bite."
No, you can't. Even though these insects suck blood, if the virus enters the mosquito, the insect does not become infected and will not regurgitate blood containing HIV into the bodies of other people.

"HIV can spread in a car crash."
There has only ever been one recorded case of HIV infection through a car accident. Blood splash transmission is extremely unlikely in any circumstances. For HIV to be passed on in a car crash, there would have to be cuts or lacerations on both people and sustained contact would have to be made—in other words, an entry and exit route for the virus. The chances of this occurring are extremely low.

"You can catch HIV having your ears pierced or getting a tattoo."
Not if you use a reputable piercer or tattooist who follows standard procedures for sterilizing equipment. The perceived risk is that needles that have been used on other people will be reused without proper sterilization, but no reputable business operates in this way. Ask a prospective piercer or tattooist if you can see the setup for sterilization: A good artist will be only too pleased to show you.

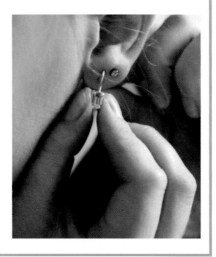

STAYING HEALTHY WITH HIV

The fact that someone has HIV does not mean that he or she will inevitably develop AIDS. The body may still have enough CD4 cells to organize fighting off infections for a long time. However, over time, as this number falls, there is a greater chance of picking up infections and the body not being able to deal with them. It is these opportunistic infections, not the HIV itself, that can cause people to become seriously ill and in some cases die.

HOW DRUGS CAN HELP THE IMMUNE SYSTEM

Combination therapy (or highly active antiretroviral therapy) is now widely available for people with HIV in the U.S., as a way of combating the virus. Combination therapy consists of different drugs (usually a cocktail of three or four drugs) that are taken every day in order to start combating the virus and preserving the number of CD4 cells that have survived the attack. These drugs are usually taken for the rest of a patient's life. This is a major undertaking that needs careful consideration. In rare cases, it may be possible to take a carefully scheduled short break from the drug regime (a structured treatment interruption), but the long term effects of this are unknown.

Side effects

Some of the drugs have unpleasant side effects and for this reason can be difficult to take. Nonetheless, it's important to take all the drugs prescribed, even if they produce feelings of nausea or fatigue.

Drug resistance

HIV is a resilient virus—it can quickly make new copies of itself and become stronger. However, as it reproduces it often makes mistakes—so each new generation, or strain, of HIV can differ from one before. This is why it is necessary to keep taking antiretroviral drugs once a course has been started—to prevent the HIV from making potentially drug-resistant copies.

Antiretroviral drug resistance can be avoided if the following guidelines are adhered to.

- At least three or four drugs should be taken in combination as advised by the clinic. If the combination is strong, the HIV virus is not able to mutate.
- The drugs must be taken exactly as prescribed. Missing doses or not taking them on time lowers the amount of drug in the body, so the virus is not properly suppressed—it

can reproduce faster and the risk of resistance increases.

- Regular viral load tests and CD4 count tests will indicate any growing drug resistance.

If resistance does develop, this usually means that the drug regimen needs to be changed.

Do antiretrovirals work?

Since it was introduced in the 1990s, combination therapy with antiretroviral drugs has helped many people with HIV. However, the drugs that suppress the HIV virus do not eliminate the virus completely from the body. Even when the levels of the virus are almost undetectable, HIV is still there and ready to replicate if given the slightest chance.

It is likely that new treatments will develop from current research based on blocking proteins or enzymes found on the HIV virus in order to prevent HIV replication and spread.

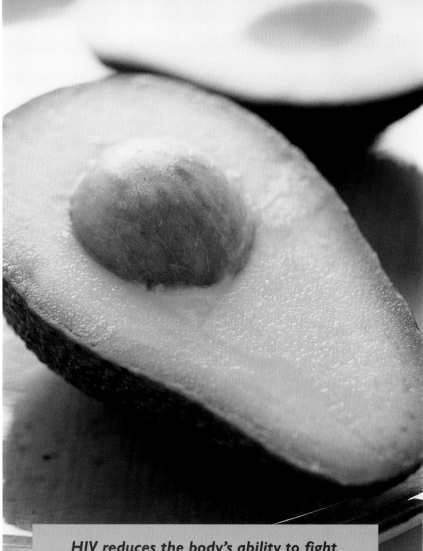

HIV reduces the body's ability to fight minor infections, so raw vegetables and fruit must be peeled or cleaned to remove hidden bacteria and germs.

Are healthcare workers at risk of HIV?

The risk of healthcare workers contracting HIV at work is low, as long as they follow safety guidelines. Casual contact with a person infected with HIV does not expose anyone—including healthcare workers—to contracting HIV. The main risk of transmission is an accidental injury from an infected needle, but this is extremely rare— scientists estimate the risk at less than 1 percent.

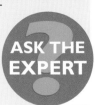

ASK THE EXPERT

WHAT CAN BE DONE TO HELP THE IMMUNE SYSTEM?

When people are ill, they are often told to eat well, drink plenty of water and get plenty of sleep. All of these things help the body fight infections; and it's the same with HIV.

- Get plenty of sleep: When the body is fatigued, it must work hard just to keep going and doesn't have time to fight infections.
- Eat a well-balanced diet: It's important to maintain a healthy weight, which may be difficult if drugs are causing sickness. Nutrient-dense foods such as

protein and carbohydrates, as well as plenty of fruit and vegetables, are recommended. Eating little and often can help if eating is a problem.

- Get regular exercise: This can also be difficult when someone is not feeling well, but exercise keeps muscles toned and improves digestion. It can also lift mood and promote good sleep.
- Manage stress: Getting too stressed can affect how the body deals with infections and how well the immune system works.
- Guard against minor infections.

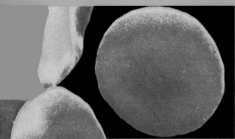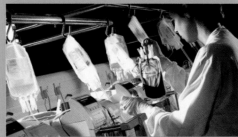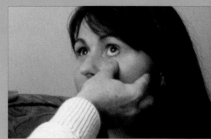

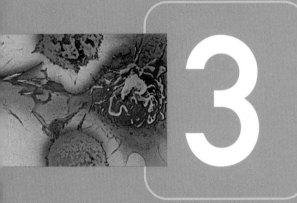

3

What happens
when things go wrong

Knowing what can go wrong

The prime causes of problems concerning the blood and immune system are infection, cancer, and genetic and hereditary factors. Another important consideration is the effect of drugs prescribed for other illnesses on the immune system.

INFECTION

Infections are a big problem when the immune system is not working well—when someone has an immune deficiency. Individuals with weakened immune systems are at higher risk of becoming infected more often and more severely than they would be if their immune systems were working normally. Bacteria and viruses that do not usually cause problems at all can result in so-called opportunistic infections, which can be life-threatening. Whatever the cause of the damage to the immune system, a patient may need treatment to prevent these opportunistic infections.

Infections can cause damage to the blood and immune system. For example, the Epstein-Barr virus not only causes infectious mononucleosis (see page 147) but may also lead to lymphoma in very few individuals. The HIV viral infection (see page 144) is well known for causing AIDS (acquired immune deficiency syndrome).

CANCER

Abnormal cells of the blood and immune system can cause cancers, such as leukemias, which affect white blood cells. These cancers tend to act differently from those affecting other organs, which usually start by forming lumps in just one part of the body and then spread to other parts. Instead, they are spread around the body by the blood from the very beginning. This may sound like very bad news, but it does mean that leukemia, for example, can be diagnosed very quickly and therefore treatment can be very effective.

PHYSICAL INJURY—TRAUMA

The most common type of injury to affect the blood circulatory system is severe bleeding or hemorrhage. Luckily, blood has evolved an effective clotting system, and in any case, the body can usually replace blood that it has lost through bleeding. Because the blood and immune system extend throughout the body, they are not vulnerable to injury in the same way as, say, an arm or a leg. An exception to this is damage to the spleen. This rather delicate organ lying in the upper left-hand side of the abdomen is relatively often damaged by accidents affecting the abdomen and because it is difficult to repair, it must sometimes be removed (see page 132).

> **The most famous carrier of an inherited blood disorder was Queen Victoria, who transmitted hemophilia to several European royal families.**

POOR NUTRITION AND OTHER DIETARY PROBLEMS

Lack of nutrients can cause blood and immune system damage. For example, a diet that does not contain very much iron or folic acid can lead to anemia. These nutrients may be lacking in a vegetarian diet, but more often, the nutrients are present in the diet at the correct

MORE COMMON

ANEMIA	LYMPHOMA	HIV (HUMAN IMMUNODEFICIENCY VIRUS)	LEUKEMIA (ALL VARIETIES)
Iron deficiency, which can lead to anemia, affects at least 3 million Americans.	About 53,000 Americans will be diagnosed with non-Hodgkin's lymphoma. Rates have nearly doubled since the 1970's.	There are 40,000 new cases in the U.S. every year. The rates are increasing among women and minorities.	Leukemia will strike about 31,000 people this year; about half of these cases will be chronic and half will be acute.
			ACUTE LEUKEMIA A vast majority of childhood leukemia is acute. The average age of a patient with acute myeloid leukemia is 65.

levels, but problems arise because the body cannot absorb enough to maintain the blood system. For example, if pernicious anemia is preventing vitamin B$_{12}$ from being absorbed, anemia will develop no matter how much vitamin B$_{12}$ is in the diet.

In other situations, the body may be using up more nutrients than it can obtain from a normal diet. For example, a woman with heavy periods may become iron deficient because of heavy bleeding. This can eventually cause iron deficiency because a normal diet will not contain enough iron to make up the deficiency. In this case the digestive system will be working flat out to absorb as much iron as it can. Taking iron tablets for a few weeks should help to relieve the anemia.

SMOKING, EXCESS ALCOHOL, AND OTHER RISKY BEHAVIORS

In addition to damaging the lining of the blood vessels, smoking increases the stickiness of platelets, which in turn increases the risk of strokes and heart attacks. Excessive alcohol consumption can harm the blood and immune system, usually through damage to other organs such as the liver. Unsafe sex (without a condom) or sharing a needle when using a hypodermic syringe allows the HIV virus to spread from one person to another.

PRESCRIBED DRUGS

Prescribed drugs frequently affect the blood and immune system. Most cytotoxic chemotherapy drugs used to treat cancer will rapidly decrease the body's ability to fight off infection. Other drugs can also affect the blood, usually in less predictable or dramatic ways. For example, aspirin and related drugs can cause a stomach ulcer. This may be so small that it does not

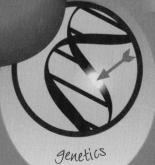

environmental pollution

infections

poor nutrition

smoking and excessive alcohol

genetics

Disorders affecting the blood and immune system
Some common and not so common diseases and disorders of the body's blood and lymph systems are listed below.

LESS COMMON

The American Cancer Society estimates that there will be 7600 new cases of Hodgkin's Disease in 2003. Death rates have fallen since the 1970's.

About 1 in 1 million people will develop SCID. Babies generally show symptoms within three months of birth.

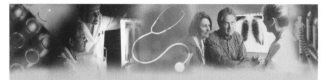

Milestones
IN MEDICINE

The first blood bank was opened in 1932 in Leningrad. Five years later, the first blood bank outside the USSR was established in Chicago by Dr. Bernard Fantus at Cook County Hospital. By setting up a hospital laboratory that could preserve and store donor blood, Fantus kick-started a movement that saw more than 1500 blood banks established in the U.S. by 1950. The American Red Cross collects over half of the blood used in transfusions in the United States, but it is not the only blood collection organization.

cause any pain, but the ulcer is constantly very slowly bleeding. This slow blood loss usually results in iron deficiency anemia.

GENETIC AND HEREDITARY FACTORS

Scientists are beginning to understand a lot more about how genes are responsible for many blood and immune system diseases. Abnormal genes can be inherited or can be mutations. Many inherited genetic diseases are described as being autosomal recessive. This means that an abnormal gene has to be inherited from each parent for the disease to be apparent in their child. Because two copies of the abnormal gene are required, these diseases tend to be rare unless parents are related to each other. Some types of severe combined immunodeficiency are inherited in this way.

Another type of inheritance is X-chromosome-linked (see page 155). If a woman inherits an X-linked disorder, she does not have its symptoms but can be a carrier and may pass the disorder on to some of her children. A man who inherits an X-linked disorder will have symptoms. Hemophilia is an example of an X-linked disorder.

Some diseases vary in severity depending on how many abnormal genes the patient has inherited. For example, having one abnormal gene for hemoglobin can cause mild sickle cell trait, but inheriting two abnormal genes causes the more severe sickle cell disease (see page 153).

In all of these examples, the abnormal gene is present in every cell in the body and will be passed on to future generations. All of these inherited disorders can be identified by genetic testing.

When mutations cause problems like leukemia or lymphoma, they are only present in the cancerous cells. The mutations are not present in egg cells or sperm cells and so cannot be passed to future generations.

AGING

The most common cancers of the blood system—chronic leukemias—occur mainly in elderly people. In general, the kind of genetic mutations that cause cancerous changes in white blood cells tend to accumulate over a person's lifetime.

ENVIRONMENTAL PROBLEMS

Problems from the environment rarely damage the blood and immune system. Very occasionally, chemicals such as lead or benzene can damage the blood system. In the past, before the amounts of lead in gasoline and paint were restricted, anemia caused by lead poisoning was relatively common in children brought up in urban environments.

As far as we know, most of the different types of radiation do not often cause damage to the blood and immune system. Powerful ionizing radiation, usually from radioactive sources, can sometimes cause cancers. Fortunately, most people are never exposed to these types of radiation.

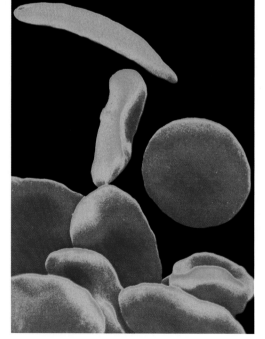

Sickle cell anemia
Sickle cell disease—characterized by sickle-shaped red blood cells—is an example of a genetically inherited disease that affects the blood. Its main symptom is anemia, which can be mild or severe.

Meet the blood and immune system experts

Because blood and lymph fluid circulate throughout the body, medical experts in diseases and disorders of the blood and immune system are not specialists in one organ, but instead treat whichever part of the body is affected.

PATHOLOGIST

Pathologists are doctors who specialize in the study of diseases. They are laboratory based and are not generally directly involved in patient care. Certain types of pathologists specialize in the study of diseases and disorders of the blood and immune systems.

- Histopathologists (also known as morbid anatomists) carry out autopsies and check samples of tissue taken by biopsy from living patients for—say—cancer.
- Microbiologists look at other samples, such as urine or sputum, to check for and identify infections; they will also recommend appropriate treatments.

Other pathologists—notably hematologists and immunologists—spend part of their time in laboratory investigations but also deal with patients face to face.

IMMUNOLOGIST

Immunologists treat patients with diseases of the immune system and run laboratory tests for diseases involving autoimmunity, immunodeficiency, and some cancers. Their work often overlaps with that carried out by allergists and rheumatologists.

ALLERGIST

Allergists are specialists who diagnose allergies and advise treatment. They help treat patients with problems ranging from rhinitis, eczema, and asthma to life-threatening allergies such as anaphylaxis.

RHEUMATOLOGIST

Rheumatologists specialize in joint diseases. These doctors manage patients with common problems such as back aches and strain injuries and also take on patients with more complex "connective tissue diseases" like rheumatoid arthritis and systemic lupus erythematosus (SLE).

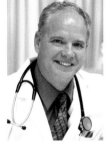

HEMATOLOGIST

Hematologists are specially trained to interpret results of investigations into diseases of the blood. They have particular expertise in looking at blood and bone marrow films.
The majority of hematologists also treat patients who suffer from disorders and diseases of the blood ranging from common conditions like anemia to complex, lifelong diseases such as hemophilia.

ONCOLOGIST AND RADIOLOGIST

Once a diagnosis has been made—probably with the assistance of a histopathologist—a cancer patient may be referred to a team of cancer specialists including an oncologist, a radiologist and a specialist surgeon as appropriate. An oncologist knows how to treat cancer with drugs. Radiologists administer radiation treatment for cancer.

BLOOD COLLECTION SERVICE

Blood collection services play an essential role in recruiting donors, ensuring that their blood is safe, and overseeing blood donations. They make sure hospitals are well supplied with blood, that it is tested and that it is stored correctly. Some also extract blood products from whole blood.

TRANSPLANT SERVICE

Transplant services facilitate the removal of organs and tissues from donors (living or dead) and the identification of the most appropriate recipient.

FINDING OUT WHAT IS WRONG

One of the first things a medical student learns is how to take a thorough patient history and do an examination following a set protocol. The history and examination can sometimes be enough to suggest a diagnosis of a blood or immunological disease. However, blood tests—and often other tests as well—are still generally required to confirm a diagnosis and to rule out other possible causes of symptoms.

Many of the tests described here can be carried out at the doctor's office. If problems are more complex, the doctor will refer the patient to a specialist, probably a hematologist or an immunologist. Tests performed by these experts generally take place in the hospital, rarely with the need for an overnight stay.

Medical history and examination

It can be helpful to make notes of symptoms before visiting the doctor to ensure that nothing is forgotten, and also to take along a list of any medications that are being taken, including dosages and timings.

TAKING A HISTORY
Obtaining an accurate patient history is an essential first step toward an accurate diagnosis.

Current complaint
The doctor will ask the patient for details of the problem. For example, if the problem is that the patient is feeling tired (possibly because of anemia), the doctor will ask how long the patient has been feeling this way, what appears to worsen the fatigue, and what alleviates it. The doctor will ask whether the patient has noticed any other symptoms—breathlessness or palpitations, for example—that may indicate anemia.

Previous medical history
The doctor will try to establish whether the patient has experienced any illnesses or irregularities in the recent or not-so-recent past that may have contributed to the current problem. For example, a doctor may ask a female patient whether she has had a series of heavy periods—a common cause of anemia.

Family history
The doctor will ask what illnesses other family members have experienced. This is important in diagnosing inherited disorders. If a parent and a brother or sister have both been anemic, for example, there is a good chance the patient has an inherited form of this condition.

Drug history
Establishing an accurate drug history is very important. This can give major clues to previous diagnoses; it also ensures that the doctor won't confuse drug side effects with symptoms of the patient's current complaint.

Aspirin and related drugs are often taken by people with aches and pains. If taken in excess, they can cause bleeding into the stomach and contribute to anemia.

Diet

Most doctors are not trained to take a thorough dietary history, but they will be able to establish, for example, whether a patient's intake of iron is too low and may be causing anemia. If a detailed dietary assessment is required, the doctor will refer the patient to a dietitian.

Sex and relationships

Because sexually transmitted diseases are so common, the doctor may ask about the patient's sexual practices and partners. Some people find this awkward, but remember that the doctor does this dozens of times a week, won't feel embarrassed, and shouldn't be shocked by anything.

The doctor also needs to ask about relationships in the patient's life. Relationships can contribute to stress and this may be relevant to the patient's physical and mental condition. In addition, the doctor may want to know whether there is a family member or friend who could take some responsibility for helping with treatment, should the need arise. For example, an elderly patient may need someone at home to help plan and monitor the taking of medication.

Occupational history

The doctor will often want to take details of employment going back many years because some occupations are associated with specific diseases. For example, chemical workers who have been exposed to benzene may be at higher risk of leukemia.

Smoking, alcohol, and recreational drug history

Because these substances can all be harmful to health, it is vital for the doctor to have honest details of whether and how much a patient smokes, drinks, or takes recreational drugs. The doctor is asking these questions for the patient's benefit and is not being judgmental. Even if a patient is doing something illegal, the conversation is confidential, and the medical profession's standards demand that anything said will not go any further.

EXAMINATION

A physical examination can be a key element in the diagnosis of many diseases and disorders of the blood and immune system. The extent of the examination depends on the symptoms—if someone has a sore throat, for example, there is generally no need to examine the whole body. Some people find a full physical examination stressful. Any patient who feels particularly uncomfortable about being examined by a doctor of the opposite sex can ask to see a doctor of the same gender instead.

General appearance and skin

A lot of information can be gained from looking at a patient's general appearance. For example, the doctor might notice that a patient has very pale skin and is lacking in energy, making anemia a possibility. If there is

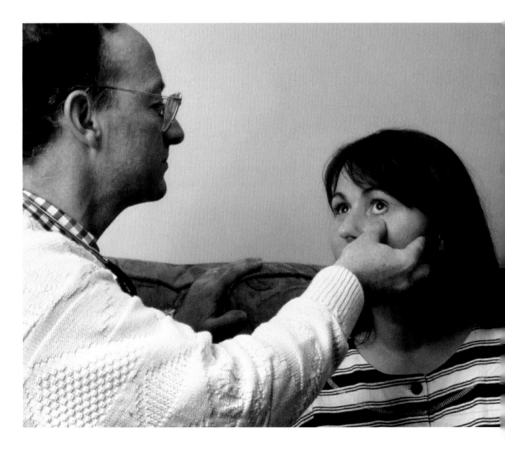

Looking for signs of anemia

A doctor examines the inside of his patient's lower eyelid for signs of anemia. A patient with anemia may have a very pale inner eyelid. In addition, the patient's skin may be much paler than usual.

bruising, bone marrow failure may be a factor. If the patient's skin has a yellow tinge (jaundice), hemolytic anemia may be suspected.

Cardiovascular system

The doctor will begin by taking the patient's pulse and blood pressure and then listening to the heart with a stethoscope. Although an infection or severe anemia can cause a fast pulse, the cardiovascular system is not usually affected by blood or immune system disorders.

Lymph nodes

When examining a patient who is being checked for cancer or infection, it is normal to check for swollen lymph glands in the locality of the disease. The doctor will check for swollen nodes in a patient's armpit if breast cancer is suspected. With some immune system and blood diseases, it is important to assess the lymph all over the body. The doctor does this by feeling for enlarged nodes in the neck, armpits, and groin. Some lymph nodes are situated deep in the chest and abdomen; these can only be assessed by CAT or MRI scanning.

Chest

The most common chest problem experienced by patients with problems with the blood or immune system is a chest infection. The doctor assesses how much air is entering the patient's chest by tapping lightly on the back or front and then listening to exactly how the breathing sounds. Although a doctor can often diagnose a chest infection by simply listening to the patient's chest and taking his or her temperature, the doctor is likely to order a chest X-ray to confirm the presence of infection.

Abdomen

For the purposes of a patient's physical examination, the mouth is regarded as the first part of the abdomen. The mouth can reveal many signs of disease—mucous membranes may look pale if the patient is anemic, for example— and the fungal infection candidosis is often seen in the mouth in cases of immune deficiency.

Nervous system

The nervous system is not often affected by blood or immune system diseases, but the doctor should make sure that everything is working normally. This is done by asking the patient to move different parts of his or her body and face in turn and then checking that the patient's ability to think and reason is as it should be.

Joints

Some blood disorders can include bleeding into the joints. In some immunological diseases—especially those affecting the connective tissue, such as systemic lupus erythematosus (SLE, see page 154) and rheumatoid arthritis—affected joints are swollen, warm, and stiff. A doctor will examine each joint in turn to establish the full extent of the problem.

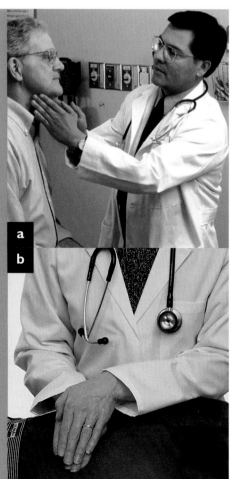

Examining the lymphatic organs

a When assessing certain blood and immune system diseases, it is important for the doctor to check the lymph throughout the body. The doctor can check for enlarged lymph nodes in the neck, armpits and groin by feeling for them. Others that are deeper in the chest and abdomen must be checked through a CT or MRI scan.
b Hematologists are especially concerned about whether the spleen —the largest lymphoid organ of all— is enlarged, which can be a sign of some types of anemia, lymphoma, or leukemia. The doctor palpates the patient's chest in order to feel the spleen—in the left upper part of the abdomen—while the patient breathes gently in and out.

Blood tests

Blood tests are very important in the diagnosis of blood and immune system disorders. Most blood tests are done either at the doctor's office or in an outpatient clinic at a hospital. The most common blood test is the complete blood count.

COMPLETE BLOOD COUNT (CBC)

In a complete blood count, an automated machine analyzes the blood sample and counts and measures each of the different cell types.

The most frequently used result from a complete blood count is the hemoglobin level. Anemia is reflected by a low level of hemoglobin. The CBC can also give information on the cause of anemia. For example, if the machine shows that red cells are small and pale, iron deficiency is the likely cause. If the red cells are larger than normal, then vitamin B_{12} or folate deficiency or alcoholic excess is likely.

Reductions in the platelet count are much less common but are seen in diseases like immune thrombocytopenia (ITP, see page 146), when bleeding can be a problem.

The white cell count is used for a variety of purposes. A raised neutrophil count is a useful clue in infections. A child with stomach pain who has a raised neutrophil count might have appendicitis, for example. If the child has a normal white cell count, the diagnosis is more likely to be a less serious problem like constipation.

Some results show a reduced neutrophil count, a condition named neutropenia. This can happen after chemotherapy and in some immunodeficiency diseases. It suggests that the patient is very vulnerable to infection and may need to take special precautions. In other

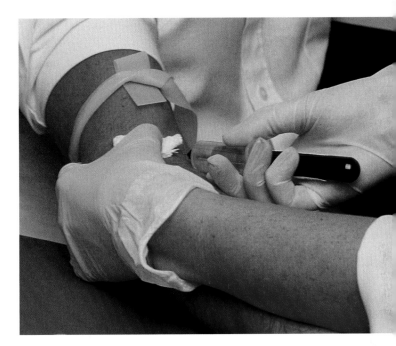

Taking a blood sample
The process of piercing a vein to remove a blood sample is called venipuncture. A strap around the upper arm compresses the arm to make the veins stand out. The blood is then drawn out of the arm by a syringe and into a container that resembles a small test tube.

situations, the blood count may show changes in the number of lymphocytes in the blood. Increased lymphocyte numbers may be the result of infection or leukemia; flow cytometry is required to distinguish between the two causes.

BLOOD FILM

In some cases, a raised white cell count can suggest problems like leukemia. In such a case, a hematologist will examine the blood through a microscope. This is done by making a blood film—spreading a very thin layer of blood onto a glass slide. The slide is processed so that each of the different cells is stained a different color.

Using a blood film, hematologists can recognize leukemic white blood cells from their unusual appearance, although flow cytometry is occasionally required to make the diagnosis.

What is measured in a complete blood count?

A complete blood count records the number, appearance, and size of the different blood cells in the sample by counting

- the red blood cells and the amount of oxygen-rich hemoglobin contained within them;
- the total number of white blood cells;
- the number of the different kinds of white blood cells, such as neutrophils and lymphocytes; and
- the platelets, which help the blood clot so that bleeding is stopped.

ASK THE EXPERT

TESTING FOR IRON, FOLATE, AND B$_{12}$

These tests investigate the cause of a patient's anemia, but they are not always the end of the story. For example, for someone with low levels of iron it would be vital to check that there is no internal bleeding. If the folate or vitamin B$_{12}$ levels are low, it becomes necessary to rule out disease of the stomach and small bowel, which could be impairing absorption of these vitamins.

BLOOD CLOTTING TESTS

These tests show whether the proteins that clot the blood are working correctly. For instance, if a sample from a boy suspected of having hemophilia (perhaps because of a family history of abnormal bleeding) was found to clot more slowly than normal, this would reinforce the suspected diagnosis. To confirm the diagnosis, it is necessary to show that the boy's factor VIII levels are low.

Checking up on anticoagulants

Much more frequently, clotting tests are used to check how well anticoagulants are working. Anticoagulants are drugs used to delay blood clotting when there has been a thrombosis (a venous thrombosis or pulmonary embolus, for example). If there has already been a blood clot, these drugs will prevent the clot from getting any bigger.

Anticoagulants can be given by injection (heparin) or by mouth (warfarin). It is very important to make sure that the drugs are working correctly. If the blood is not anticoagulated enough, there is a risk of more clotting. If the blood is anticoagulated too much, there will be a risk of bleeding. Patients respond differently to the same dose of anticoagulants, and other factors can destabilize expected results. For example, a course of antibiotics can either increase or decrease clotting ability.

For these reasons, patients on anticoagulants need regular clotting tests, usually every month or so. If the clotting test results have changed, a doctor may recommend changing the dose of anticoagulant.

THYROID FUNCTION TESTS

Thyroid function tests are blood tests that measure the amount of thyroxine and are used to diagnose this group of diseases. Thyroid function tests are also used to monitor patients with thyroid disease once they are receiving treatment. The thyroid gland secretes a hormone called thyroxine, which has widespread effects on the metabolism of the whole body. The thyroid can secrete

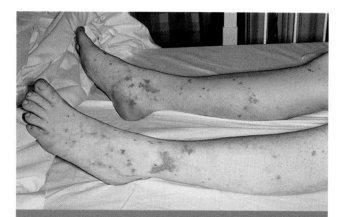

Clotting tests and meningococcal septicemia
Sometimes people with serious injuries or infections can begin to have problems with blood clotting. An example is meningococcal septicemia. This causes small bruises in the skin because the bacteria causing the infection trigger abnormal clotting. This depletes the amount of clotting proteins available, and bleeding elsewhere can become a problem. In this case, clotting test results will be abnormal.

too much thyroxine, resulting in hyperthyroidism, for example in Graves' disease, or too little thyroxine, causing hypothyroidism, as in Hashimoto's disease.

COOMBS' TEST

In Coombs' test, or the antiglobulin test, a sample of blood taken from a patient is examined to find out whether the patient's red cells are being attacked by antibodies. This happens if blood of an incorrect group is transfused into a patient. Sometimes it can happen because the immune system attacks the body's own cells—a condition known as autoimmune hemolytic anemia (see page 143). Coombs' test could be used in either of these situations.

HEMOGLOBIN ELECTROPHORESIS

Some people inherit abnormal genes for hemoglobin, the red pigment in the red blood cells that carries oxygen from lungs to the tissues. If the hemoglobin is abnormal, the red cells can become damaged and even destroyed, causing types of anemia. The two common forms are sickle cell disease and thalassemia. These are diagnosed by hemoglobin electrophoresis. Electrophoresis is a process for distinguishing between slightly different proteins; in this case, it distinguishes between normal and abnormal hemoglobin.

FLOW CYTOMETRY

Flow cytometers fire lasers at each cell in a blood sample and collect data on how the laser beam is bounced back to a light detector. A flow cytometer can look at several thousand white cells in a few seconds and distinguish each of them on the basis of subtle differences in size, how granular they are, and different molecules on the surface of the cells. This type of counting could not possibly be done by humans looking through microscopes, and many advances in immunology and hematology have resulted from this technology. Flow cytometers can count even tiny numbers of abnormal cells mixed in with the normal cells.

Advantages of flow cytometry over blood film

In many cases, it is possible for hematologists or immunologists to find what they are looking for by examining the different populations of white cells on a blood film. However, some of the different populations look the same under the microscope. For instance, the different populations of lymphocytes—helper T cells, B cells, and cytotoxic cells—may all appear identical. In some situations, it is necessary to distinguish among and count these different cells.

For example, an increase in the number of lymphocytes that show up in a blood count may be the result of infection or may reflect leukemia. If there is an infection, it is normal for a mixed population of B cells and helper T cells to cause the increase in the number of lymphocytes, and each cell will be different from all the others. In leukemia, the lymphocytes will all be the daughter cells of one single cancerous cell. This means that all the lymphocytes will, for example, be B cells, and each one will have identical molecules on its surface. Flow cytometry is the only

Flow cytometry

A technician uses a flow cytometer to analyze a blood sample. The blood cells have been tagged with a fluorescent antibody that binds to certain types of cells. The cells are then passed in single file through a beam of light, which causes tagged cells to fluoresce so that they can be counted on a detector.

way of making the leukemia diagnosis in this situation. After a patient has had treatment for leukemia, flow cytometry is used to check whether the cancerous cells have been completely cleared. Even if only 1 in 10,000 lymphocytes in the blood was cancerous, it would be possible for this one cell to reproduce itself, causing a return of the leukemia once treatment has stopped.

Monitoring HIV infections

HIV infection damages the immune system by destroying the helper T cells. This damage happens gradually over several years. Patients with HIV do not need treatment unless there are high levels of HIV in the blood—detected by polymerase chain reaction (PCR), see page 109—or if the helper T cell count has become low. Flow cytometry is the only way of accurately counting the number of helper cells in the blood. Helper T cells are distinguished from other cells by having a high level of a molecule called CD4 on their surface. Flow cytometers count the number of cells with CD4 on the surface, so the helper T cell count is sometimes referred to as the CD4 count.

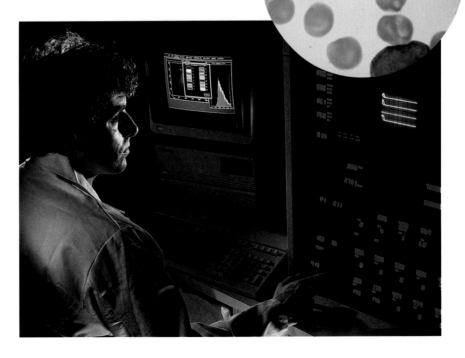

This blood film *shows three myeloblast cells, which indicate acute myeloblastic leukemia.*

Bone marrow tests

There are two important bone marrow tests: the bone marrow aspirate, in which liquid bone marrow is sucked out with a needle, and the bone marrow biopsy, in which a core of solid bone is taken.

Bone marrow tests are often much more useful than blood films for explaining the reason behind a blood problem. This is because bone marrow is the place where the red blood cells, platelets, and most white blood cells are manufactured, and so by examining the bone marrow, it is possible to inspect the blood manufacturing process.

WHAT ARE THEY USED FOR?

In a patient with a low platelet count, for example, the doctor can tell from a marrow sample whether the blood manufacturing process is working. If platelets are not being produced, this can cause a low platelet count (bone marrow failure). If platelets are being produced, they must be being destroyed elsewhere in the body (as in the spleen in immune thrombocytopenia, see page 146).

The most serious problems with manufacturing white cells are leukemia and lymphoma. Bone marrow tests are particularly useful in diagnosing these diseases.

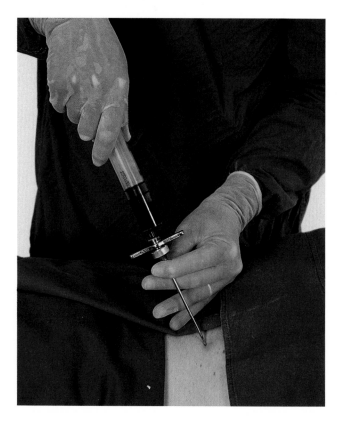

HOW ARE THEY DONE?

Both procedures can be done in an outpatient clinic in about half an hour: Adults do not have to be admitted to the hospital. Small children usually have bone marrow tests done under general anesthetic.

Both tests begin by cleaning the skin with a disinfectant such as iodine. Next, the doctor will inject a local anesthetic into the skin. This takes a few seconds to work. Because the procedures aim to take samples from the middle of the bones, the next step is to anesthetize the bone itself. Bone is very sensitive to pain, so injecting local anesthetic into the bone is likely to be painful for the first few seconds.

Bone marrow aspirate

The aspirate can be taken from the iliac crest (the back of the pelvic bones) or the sternum (the breastbone). A wide bore needle is inserted into the middle of the bone, and the semiliquid marrow is sucked out into a syringe. Very often, a bone marrow aspirate is all that is needed.

Bone marrow biopsy

The biopsy is usually taken from the iliac crest. Undergoing the bone marrow biopsy procedure is more uncomfortable than the aspirate because it takes a core of bone marrow and solid bone. This is most useful when doctors want to look at how cells are arranged in the bone marrow, which is not possible with a liquid sample. Cancer and some hematological problems can only be diagnosed by doing a biopsy.

After the procedure

Once the procedure is complete, a patient is requested to lie down for an hour or so before going home. When the local anesthetic wears off, the patient may feel a dull ache at the site where the sample was taken.

Taking a sample of bone marrow aspirate
Semiliquid bone marrow—the aspirate—is sucked out into a syringe from a puncture made into the back of the patient's pelvis. The aspiration is done to test the functioning of the patient's marrow.

Breakthroughs in genetic testing

The mapping of the human genome—the 23 pairs of chromosomes that make up each cell in the human body—has triggered major advances in medical research. Among disorders of the blood and immune system, genetic testing has improved diagnosis of leukemia and HIV infection.

CYTOGENETIC ANALYSIS

There are 22 pairs of identical chromosomes and one pair of sex chromosomes in every normal cell. Cytogenetic testing is a way of checking that chromosomes are not damaged. It is especially important in two situations:

- Testing for chronic myeloid leukemia In some people, chromosomes are damaged and genes become mixed up. This can lead to leukemia. For example, a damaged chromosome (the "Philadelphia chromosome") occurs often in chronic myeloid leukemia. Cytogenetic testing for the Philadelphia chromosome is both a diagnostic test and a way of measuring response to treatment.

- Prenatal testing for Down's syndrome before birth In some genetic diseases, chromosomes are damaged in very specific ways. In Down's syndrome, there are three copies of chromosome number 21. Because only a few cells are needed to carry out cytogenetic testing, tiny samples of the fluid surrounding a fetus can be tested for cells with an extra chromosome 21 to check for Down's syndrome before birth.

Polymerase chain reaction in action
In this technique, the DNA of a single cell treated with polymerase enzymes is induced to replicate many times. This enables amplification of DNA in sufficient quantities to facilitate genetic analysis. Many recent advances in cancer diagnosis, HIV treatment, gene therapy, and the Human Genome Project would not have been possible without the invention of PCR.

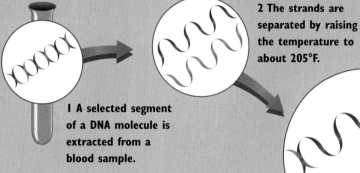

1 A selected segment of a DNA molecule is extracted from a blood sample.

2 The strands are separated by raising the temperature to about 205°F.

3 Synthetic DNA fragments are then added, with the temperature at 125°F. These bind to the two DNA strands.

POLYMERASE CHAIN REACTION (PCR)

Using the PCR method of replicating sequences of DNA in a test tube, scientists are now able to read the sequence of DNA for any given gene more rapidly than ever before, and this has been put to a number of uses.

- PCR can detect DNA mutations known to cause cancer or leukemia. This is a useful diagnostic test for some cancers.

- PCR technologies can detect one leukemia cell or cancer cell among a million normal cells. This means that it can detect a recurrence of the disease after treatment much earlier than other tests.

- By measuring the precise amount of HIV (human immunodeficiency virus) in infected patients' blood, PCR helps specialists decide the best time to start anti-HIV treatments. These "viral load" tests are used with helper T cell (CD4) counts.

4 The enzyme DNA polymerase is added, and with the temperature at about 160°F, an exact copy of the original DNA segment is created.

5 By repeatedly raising and lowering the temperature of the DNA strands, many copies are produced rapidly.

Antibody and allergy testing

An antigen is a substance—usually a protein—that the body regards as dangerous. To counteract the danger, the body produces a special kind of blood protein called an antibody that circulates in the plasma, seeking to attack the antigen and render it harmless.

ELISA TESTING

An enzyme-linked immunosorbent assay (ELISA) test measures whether antibodies will bind onto a specific antigen. These tests are most often used to diagnose infection. During an infection, the immune system normally produces antibodies against the responsible virus or bacteria. It is usually much easier to diagnose infection by looking for antibodies than by looking for the virus or bacteria. Blood collection services use ELISA to check donated blood for antibodies against viral infections such as HIV and hepatitis B and C.

AUTOANTIBODY TESTS

Autoantibody tests are used to help diagnose autoimmune diseases. The tests work by seeing whether the patient's blood contains antibodies that bind to normal healthy body tissues. For example, in pernicious anemia,

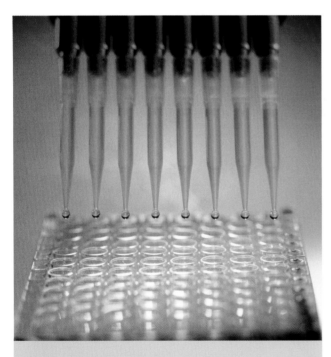

ELISA antibody test

Multi-pipettes are suspended over a multi-well sample tray in an ELISA test. To measure the amount of a target substance in the blood, an antibody that binds with the target substance is mixed with the blood sample.

autoantibodies are produced that bind to the stomach-lining cells that normally help the body to absorb vitamin B_{12}.

POLYMORPHISMS AND FORENSIC TESTING

Each individual has a group of human leukocyte antigens (HLA), DNA, and proteins that is almost unique. Some people may have relatively common HLA genes; others may share their HLA genes with just one in every few thousand other people. These genetic differences among people are called polymorphisms.

Establishing paternity

Testing to identify genetic polymorphisms has been used in paternity cases, although strictly speaking, genetic fingerprinting can rule out a potential father but cannot completely confirm one. If a child shares polymorphisms with the suspected father, he could have inherited them from him. If the man and child share no polymorphisms, then the man couldn't possibly be the father.

Forensic testing

DNA is very stable—even material from the ancient Egyptian tombs of the pharaohs can be used to identify family trees. This characteristic makes genetic finger prints useful in criminal investigations. Tiny traces of DNA—for example, on a cigarette butt being used as a piece of evidence—can rule suspects out or in.

IMMUNOGLOBULIN AND PLASMA ELECTROPHORESIS

Immunoglobulins are structurally related proteins that act as antibodies. They are produced by the immune system and normally bind onto bacteria or viruses and destroy them. In autoimmune diseases, antibodies are produced that bind onto normal components of the body and cause disease rather than help protect the body from it.

Very high levels of immunoglobulins are also produced in some tumors, such as those associated with myeloma and lymphoma. Compared with normal antibodies produced in response to an infection, the immunoglobulins produced by tumor cells all have identical structures because they originate from one original cancerous cell. These identical cells and immunoglobulins are sometimes described as monoclonal. In myeloma (see page 150), monoclonal immunoglobulins are found in the blood and in the urine.

How electrophoresis helps

Electrophoresis is a technique in which electrically charged particles in solution (sometimes a serum or plasma) are separated into bands by having an electric current passed through them. Electrophoresis shows whether immunoglobulins are monoclonal. It can also show if levels of immunoglobulins are very low, which would indicate antibody deficiencies. People with low levels of immunoglobulin are very prone to recurring chest and sinus infection. Immunoglobulin treatment can prevent infections from getting worse.

ALLERGY TESTING

Allergy testing aims to identify the substances to which a patient is allergic. The particular substances to which an individual is allergic—for example, peanuts, pollen, or dust mites—are referred to as allergens. Most allergies result in irritating symptoms, but some can be debilitating, and in its most serious form—known as anaphylaxis—an allergic reaction can be life-threatening.

Safeguards in place before testing

Allergy tests should be carried out by either a medically trained allergist or by a doctor with expertise in chest medicine, dermatology, or pediatrics. The tests can be dangerous—there is always a chance of provoking an extreme anaphylactic reaction. For this reason, there must always be resuscitation equipment and experienced, well-trained staff on hand.

There are three well-established tests for allergies. It should be kept in mind that test results are not always 100 percent accurate, especially in the case of skin and

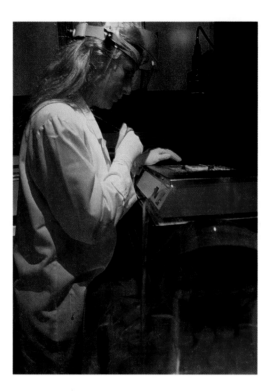

Electrophoresis in action
A laboratory technician is separating particles within a gel so that they form distinct bands. This is done by applying an electric field to the particles. The particles may be proteins, such as immunoglobulins, or DNA fragments. Normal or fluorescent dyes may be used to view the particles, or they may be labeled with radioisotopes.

challenge testing; the results may not actually reflect the true clinical situation.

Skin test

This is done by injecting a tiny amount of allergen into the outer layer of the skin. Within a few minutes, a patient who is truly allergic to the allergen will experience an itchy swelling up to ½ inch in diameter on the surface of the skin. The itchiness may last as long as a couple of hours. Very rarely, there can be a more serious reaction, especially if the patient has a history of anaphylaxis. Substances that are harmless for an individual cause no swelling at all. If the patient is on antihistamine tablets, the tests may not work.

Challenge test

This is usually done to test for the cause of a suspected food allergy. In the safe environment of the clinic, the patient eats a tiny amount of the suspected allergen, usually made up into a cookie or cracker. The reactions to the food can then be noted.

Allergy blood tests

Sometimes called specific IgE tests or RAST (radioallergosorbent) tests, allergy blood tests aim to show how much of the allergy-causing antibody—the IgE—a patient has that will act against a specific allergen.

Allergy blood tests are much less reliable than skin testing. They are reserved for situations when skin testing is unsafe (where there is a history of anaphylaxis or eczema or in very young children) or when the patient has been taking antihistamines.

CURRENT TREATMENTS

Medical help is at hand for a wide range of conditions affecting the blood and immune system. More sophisticated drugs than ever before are available for the control and treatment of diseases and disorders. Doctors use chemotherapy and radiation to treat cancers of the blood and lymphatic systems; after cancer treatment, stem cell transplantation is available if needed to repair a patient's damaged bone marrow cells. A recent major breakthrough is stem cell gene therapy—used to treat severe combined immunodeficiency (SCID) in children.

Drugs for blood and the immune system

Drugs are used not only to treat the causes of diseases and disorders of the blood and immune system but also the adverse side effects of other treatments.

AN OVERVIEW OF PRESCRIBED DRUG USE

Drugs help treat diseases and disorders of the blood and immune system in many different ways.

- There are drugs that stop unwanted blood clotting and also drugs that help to clot the blood.
- A primary weapon in the fight against cancers of the blood is the use of drugs in chemotherapy. These drugs kill as many cancerous blood cells as possible —but healthy cells are also destroyed, meaning almost inevitably that a patient's ability to fight off infection is seriously impaired. Antibiotics are often prescribed to help patients while their immune systems recover. Interferons are also prescribed to inhibit tumor cells.
- Drugs are used to suppress the automatic attempts of the body's immune system to reject a "foreign" organ that has been transplanted into the body and also after stem cell transplantation.
- Drugs also help fight immunosuppressive diseases, as with drugs prescribed to combat HIV infection.

Drugs used for treating HIV infection

The goal of drug therapy against HIV infection (see page 144) is to increase the length and quality of life by improving immune function. This is achieved by reducing the amount of replicating virus to as low a level as possible for as long as possible in all sites where HIV-infected cells are present, thereby preventing infection of new cells and further damage to the immune system. There are currently three classes of anti-HIV drugs in use in the United States. They are often prescribed in combination with each other.

NRIs (NUCLEOSIDE TRANSCRIPTASE INHIBITORS) NRI zidovudine (AZT) was the first anti-HIV drug. NRIs are generally well tolerated, but side effects can include nausea and fatigue.

PIs (PROTEASE INHIBITORS) A dramatic decline in the clinical progression of HIV disease and HIV-related deaths followed the introduction of PIs in 1996. There are many tablets to take, and there may be adverse side effects; PIs can't be taken with some common prescription drugs, such as antihistamines and the oral contraceptive pill, or with some foods.

NNRTIs (NON-NUCLEOSIDE REVERSE TRANSCIOTASE INHIBITORS) Resistance to these drugs develops quickly, but they are a lot simpler to take than PIs; there may be adverse side effects such as drowsiness or rashes.

Drugs that prevent blood clotting

Drugs taken to prevent the blood from clotting are most often given following surgery, during kidney dialysis, or to patients who are naturally at risk of forming blood clots inside blood vessels. These drugs can be taken by mouth or injection.

Blood clots usually form as a response to injury. When a clot forms for some other reason, there is a risk that it might become lodged in a blood vessel and even block the blood supply to the heart or brain. There are two sorts of drugs that doctors prescribe to stop abnormal blood clotting: anticoagulants and antiplatelet drugs.

Drugs given by injection take immediate effect; taken by mouth, they will work after a few days. The effect of anticoagulants and antiplatelet drugs can be enhanced or reduced by other drugs and illnesses, so patients must keep their doctors informed of any changes in their health or medication. People taking such drugs orally over the long term should carry a card that outlines their treatment.

Are drugs ever taken to encourage blood clotting—and thereby stop bleeding?

When bleeding is difficult to stop—such as after surgery—clotting can be encouraged by using an antifibrinolytic such as tranexamic acid. This drug can also be given to hemophiliacs before dental surgery and other minor operations. Severe bleeding in hemophiliacs may be treated by injecting into the blood a concentrated form of the factor VIII that is missing.

ASK THE EXPERT?

ANTICOAGULANTS

These drugs reduce the effectiveness of the coagulation factors within the blood that promote blood clotting; which factors are affected varies from drug to drug. The two most commonly used drugs are heparin and warfarin.

- Heparin is given by injection and acts rapidly but is only effective for a short time. It is used in hospitals during or after surgery to prevent clot formation and during kidney dialysis to prevent clots from forming in dialysis machines. Heparin can also stabilize existing clots so that fragments don't break off and travel to other parts of the body. Lengthy operations—especially those involving the pelvis, hips, or knees—can lead to deep venous thrombosis (DVT). Low doses of heparin reduce the incidence of DVT and fatal embolism in patients undergoing general surgery by 60–70 percent.

  Too much heparin can cause bleeding, which is why treatment has to be carefully supervised. Newer versions of heparin, called low-molecular-weight heparins (dalteparin, enoxaparin, and tinzaparin) are longer-lasting and need less monitoring.

- Warfarin, commonly known as Coumadin, is the most widely used oral anticoagulant. It is generally taken long-term as a preventative treatment for patients at risk of a stroke, heart attack, or disturbed heart rhythms (atrial fibrillation) or who have an artificial heart valve. It interferes with vitamin-K-dependent synthesis of clotting factors. Its use is monitored in regular blood tests at the start of treatment to measure its effect on clotting time. The dosage is adjusted during this phase. Bleeding is the main side effect of oral anticoagulants, and doctors will have an emergency plan in the event of bleeding.

ANTIPLATELET DRUGS

Antiplatelet drugs prevent clots forming by binding to platelets in the blood and lessening their ability to stick together and form clots.

- Aspirin helps thin the blood and is taken long-term in low doses by many people at risk of blood clots in the blood circulatory system or of stroke, heart attack, angina, or atherosclerosis.
- Dipyridamole can be taken in combination with aspirin to reduce the risk of a second stroke. This drug dilates the blood vessels and inhibits platelets.
- Clopidogrel is taken to help prevent heart attacks and strokes. It can also be taken with aspirin; the two together have been shown to be more effective than aspirin alone.

THROMBOLYTIC AGENTS

These are used to dissolve clots already in existence. The most common thrombolytics (also known as fibrinolytics) are streptokinase and alteplase.

Treating anemia

The word anemia comes from the Ancient Greek for "lack of blood." Medically, the term is used to indicate a shortage of hemoglobin—the oxygen-carrying protein in red blood cells. Treatments for this common condition vary depending on the cause.

FINDING THE CAUSE

Whether a patient is anemic can be settled quickly and easily by means of a blood test. A low level of hemoglobin in the blood indicates anemia. Effective treatment of anemia, however, depends on establishing its precise cause. So before treatment can begin, further tests are necessary to find the exact mechanism responsible. For example, initial tests may show that the cause is iron deficiency, but then the doctor must determine why the body has run out of iron. Tests can include bone marrow aspiration (see page 108), and genetic testing, X-rays and other imaging scans to pick up problems affecting organs such as the stomach, intestines, liver, or kidneys.

Once the cause of the anemia has been diagnosed, treatment can be decided upon and commenced. Treatments range from simply taking iron tablets once a day or vitamin B_{12} injections every month to complex operations, such as a splenectomy for autoimmune hemolytic anemia (see page 143).

Eat to beat anemia

Anemia caused by a diet deficient in iron or folate can be treated with an iron and folate-rich diet or iron and folic acid supplements. These dietary changes may also help with anemia caused by regular loss of blood.

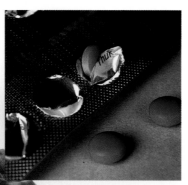

Anemia caused by iron deficiency

A low hemoglobin count caused by lack of iron is the most common cause of anemia. The two main reasons are loss of iron through slow, chronic bleeding (heavy periods are a common cause of anemia) or (less commonly) an iron-deficient diet. Slow intermittent internal bleeding, such as from a gastric or duodenal ulcer, can be stopped by surgery. Blood transfusions are rarely given just to treat anemia.

Anemia from vitamin B_{12} deficiency

Anemia resulting from vitamin B_{12} deficiency is rarely caused by poor diet alone, unless the patient's diet is very restricted. The problem generally lies in the body's inability to absorb vitamin B_{12} and is controlled by regular injections of vitamin B_{12}.

Anemia resulting from bone marrow failure

Bone marrow can fail to make or sustain a sufficient number of red blood cells because of cancer or as an aftereffect of cancer treatment such as chemotherapy. In this case, the treatment is generally stem cell transplants into the bone marrow (see page 120).

Anemia from genetic disorders

There are genetic blood disorders that lead to abnormalities within hemoglobin molecules. The two most common are thalassemia (see page 154) and anemia from sickle cell disease (see page 153).

In the case of thalassemia, the standard treatment is regular blood transfusions. Sickle cell anemia is best tackled by means of antibiotics and folic acid taken on a regular basis. In a sickle cell crisis—a flare-up of the disease—a blood transfusion may be needed.

Hemolytic anemia

Hemolytic anemia occurs when red blood cells break down prematurely. There are different causes, and the treatment options vary according to the cause (see page 142).

Blood transfusions

A patient needs a blood transfusion when blood is being lost at such a rate that the body can't make up the loss on its own—common causes are accidental injury or surgery. Occasionally, a transfusion is ordered to treat anemia that won't respond to other medicines.

Before recommending a blood transfusion or treatment with blood products, doctors need to make a risk assessment. This means that the doctor must balance the possible benefits of a transfusion against the potential risks. For example, someone who is bleeding because he or she has just been hit by a bus may well need a life-saving blood transfusion. The tiny risk of infection is overwhelmed by the serious effects of the hemorrhage.

WHAT CAN GO WRONG

- **Infection** A patient may become infected with a blood-borne virus during the blood transfusion process. This is now very rare, thanks to the tests done on blood donors before they give blood (see page 55).
- **Blood mismatch** A patient may be given blood of the wrong type. If this happens, antibodies in the recipient's blood will attack the donated cells and destroy them. To prevent this, not only is the patient's blood type carefully established, but, as a second check, a sample of the patient's antibodies in serum is mixed with blood cells belonging to the donor; this is called a cross-match. Units of blood identified by this test as safe for the recipient are then labeled and held in a refrigerator until needed. Then, just before the unit of blood is transfused, two nurses read off the patient's name, date of birth, and hospital number from the label and confirm that the blood is going to the right person.

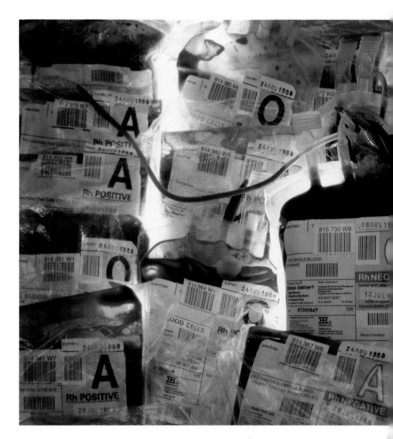

Bags of blood
Donated blood awaits collection at a blood collection center. Blood is classified as A, B, AB, or O and as Rhesus (Rh) positive or negative. A, B, and O are different molecules that the immune system of the recipient of a blood transfusion may recognize as foreign.

- **Feverish reactions** A patient may develop a fever during a transfusion because the immune system recognizes proteins in the donated blood. The fever is usually mild.

BLOOD PRODUCTS FOR TRANSFUSION

Donated blood is either left whole or separated into red blood cells, platelets, and plasma. The blood is spun (centrifuged) at high speed to separate it into red blood cells and plasma. Then, if necessary, the plasma is spun to draw out the platelets. Most transfusions that take place use whole blood or red blood cells suspended in a special nutrient solution.

ON THE CUTTING EDGE

One blood type for all

Scientists at the New York Blood Center are trying to create a "universal" donor blood for transfusion to do away with the problem of patients needing compatible blood. So far, they have managed to convert type B blood into type O, and this is now being used in clinical trials. They are also well on the way to being able to convert type A blood to type O (a more complicated procedure) and to remove the rhesus factor.

Platelet transfusions

Platelets are tiny packets of cytoplasm that play a crucial role in the blood-clotting process (see page 24). They are given to people with dangerously low platelet counts, such as those suffering from the platelet disorder immune thrombocytopenic purpura (ITP) or bone marrow failure (see page 138). Donations from several different people are usually required to give a patient enough platelets.

Plasma transfusions

Plasma is a solution of proteins. Whole plasma is given to
• patients with conditions such as serious burns or infections to try to restore their damaged blood-clotting mechanism; and
• patients who have problems with low blood pressure.
Plasma is also broken down—known as fractionated— to produce different proteins including
• factor VIII, for hemophilia;
• albumen, sometimes given to people in shock;
• anti D antibody, for hemolytic disease of the newborn; and
• immunoglobulin, for antibody-deficient patients.
Some of these proteins are present in plasma only in small amounts. Plasma from hundreds, even thousands, of donors is mixed in order to yield enough proteins and to make the fractionation process economical. A problem with mixing or "pooling" plasma from many donors is the increased risk of the finished product carrying blood-borne infection. The risk of infection with hepatitis or HIV from plasma is now very low because of donor screening.

From donor to freezer
After blood has been donated at a collection center, it is sent to a blood bank where it is processed before storage. A technician is shown here setting up automated extraction of plasma from donated blood. After separation, the plasma is frozen until needed.

SCREENING BLOOD DONORS

Donors are asked questions about the risk of infection before they are allowed to give blood. Each blood donation is then tested for HIV, hepatitis, and other infections. Plasma and fractionated products undergo further treatments to ensure that they are safe. For example, they may be heat treated so that doctors are as certain as they can be that any viruses that have escaped the testing process have been removed.

At the moment, blood donors can't be tested for variant Creutzfeldt-Jakob disease (vCJD), which is thought to spread from mad cow disease and could theoretically spread through plasma products. To reduce this risk, blood from UK donors is not fractionated. All the fractionation taking place in the UK, where mad cow was a problem, is done using plasma imported from overseas. The U.S. government has taken things a step further. They have told their transfusion services that people who have visited the UK for long periods should not be allowed to donate blood at all.

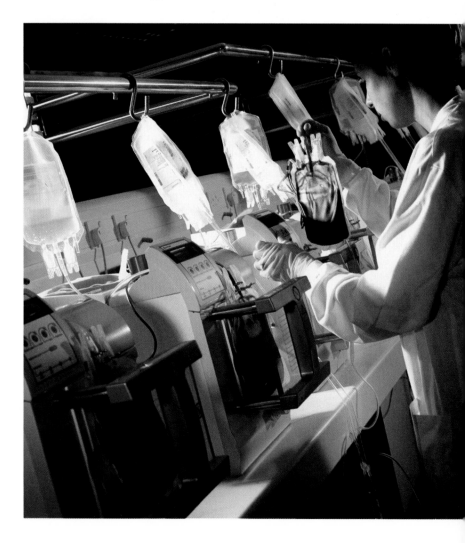

Drug treatments for cancers of the blood

When the body is fighting cancers of the blood and the immune system, its first line of attack is generally the use of drugs to kill as many cancer cells as possible. Antibiotics also come into play to combat the patient's susceptibility to infection after chemotherapy.

CHEMOTHERAPY

Chemotherapy is a term associated with administration of drugs as a method of cancer treatment. The drugs used to kill cancer cells are also called cytotoxics.

Chemotherapy is used to treat various cancers affecting the blood and immune systems. All cells, whether normal or cancerous, go through phases of growth and development during their life cycles. Chemotherapy drugs interfere with the cellular activities during one or more of these phases. The drugs circulate in the blood to achieve a total body (systemic) effect.

The choice of chemotherapy for each patient depends on the type and location of the cancer, its stage of development, and the general health of the patient. In most cases, the dose is calculated from the height and weight of the patient and is given by mouth, injection, or through a special intravenous line. It is standard practice to administer a combination of drugs, each exerting different effects and acting on specific stages of the cell cycle. At the same time, combining drugs reduces the chance of drug resistance developing.

Malignant cells have a less effective repair capacity than normal cells, so chemotherapy is given intermittently rather than at a constant low dose; this gives the healthy cells a chance to recover. The length and frequency of chemotherapy depends on the type of cancer, the drugs being used, and how the patient responds to them; and drugs can be given daily, weekly, or monthly. A cycle is established, with the next treatment occurring once the normal stem cells have had enough time to recover from the last. Sometimes treatment is given in an on-and-off cycle that includes rest periods so the body has a chance to build healthy new cells and regain strength. Drugs known as growth factors are now available to accelerate the body's recovery of blood cell production.

Possible side effects

One of the main problems with chemotherapy is that normal cells are killed in addition to cancer cells. Side effects depend on which normal cells are affected.

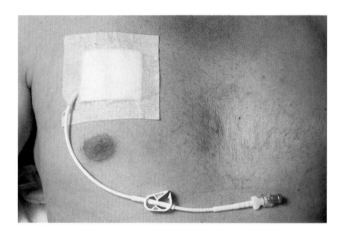

Venous access through a Hickman catheter
A patient receiving chemotherapy over a period of months needs a long-term venous access device. A Hickman catheter made of silicone rubber allows chemotherapy to be given into a large central vein (the vena cava) or directly into the right atrium of the heart.

- Bone marrow damage can lead to infections and bleeding, which is overcome by antibiotics and platelets.
- Damage to the gastrointestinal tract can cause a sore mouth, nausea, and diarrhea.
- Damage to hair follicles can cause temporary hair loss.
- Damage to the reproductive organs can cause infertility, but both eggs and sperm can be frozen.

TARGETED TREATMENT WITH MONOCLONAL ANTIBODIES

Monoclonal antibodies are a new class of drugs specially designed to recognize malignant cells, bind to them, and destroy them. An anti-CD20 antibody (rituximab) is active against lymphoma cells, anti-CD33 antibody works against acute myeloid leukemia cells, and anti-CD52 fights chronic lymphocytic leukemia cells. Targeting the attack on cancerous cells cuts down on many of the adverse effects of broad-based chemotherapy treatments, which damage healthy cells in addition to cancerous ones. Unfortunately, there may still be side effects such as rash, fever, and shivering. Also, anti-CD20 and anti-CD52 antibodies can impair the immune system, increasing the risk of viral infections.

Drugs for treating cancers associated with blood and the immune system

Some of the drugs currently being used to treat hematological cancers are listed below. The drugs mostly work by inhibiting DNA synthesis or damaging DNA, thereby preventing cells from growing and dividing. Side effects vary, with some patients experiencing fewer side effects than others. In addition to the side effects listed, almost all the drugs reduce blood-cell production by bone mar resulting in a low blood count and often leading to infection, anemia and bleeding; other common side effects are nausea and hair

Drug name	Drug type	Used to treat	Possible adverse effects
methotrexate (MTX)	antimetabolite	lymphomas; acute lymphoblastic leukemia; meningeal leukemia	mucositis (inflammation of gastrointestinal diarrhea; liver damage; lung problems
cytosine arabinoside (Ara-C)	antimetabolite	acute myeloid leukemia	poor appetite; sore mouth; slurred speech, gait; conjunctivitis; liver damage; gastrointesti
6-mercaptopurine, 6-thioguannine	purine analog antimetabolite	6-MP: acute lymphoblastic leukemia 6-TG: chronic myeloid leukemia	loss of appetite; sore mouth; liver damage
vincristine (Oncovin), vinblastine	vinca alkaloids	acute leukemias; lymphomas	tingling and numbness of fingers and toes; muscular weakness
bleomycin	cytotoxic antibiotic	Hodgkin's disease; lymphomas	lung fibrosis; skin toxicity (redness, pigmen ulceration); fever and malaise
cyclophosphamide	alkylating agent	various hematological malignancies	bladder damage
doxorubicin, daunorubicin	anthracyclines	various hematological malignancies	mucositis; damage to heart if taken in exce
L-asparaginase	enzyme	lymphoid malignancies	problems with blood clotting more or less easily than before
dexamethasone, prednisolone	steroids	lymphoid malignancies	fluid retention; high blood pressure; diabet increased appetite; infection; osteoporosis
all-trans retinoic acid (ATRA)	derived from vitamin A	acute promyelocytic leukemia	dry skin; abnormal liver function; fluid in lu

ANTIBIOTICS AFTER CHEMOTHERAPY

A patient's white blood cell count can be affected by chemotherapy, leaving the patient vulnerable to infection during treatment. A very low white cell count is known as neutropenia (see page 146). The blood count is at its lowest 10 to 14 days following chemotherapy treatment, but the acute immunosuppressive effects of most drugs used in chemotherapy do not extend for prolonged periods beyond the time of active drug administration.

One of the main symptoms of infection is a high temperature; if this occurs, a patient should contact the doctor immediately, because antibiotics will be needed. Aggressive antibiotic therapy using antibiotics such as gentamicin, ceftazidime, and vancomycin has greatly aided the treatment of infectious complications.

Some patients take an antibiotic called co-trimoxazole during treatment and for a while afterward, to prevent a common lung infection, called pneumocystis, to which immunosuppressed patients are susceptible.

INTERFERON

Interferons are substances (produced by white blood cells and artificially in the laboratory) prescribed to patients to inhibit tumor cells from growing inside the body. Interferon alpha is able to slow tumor growth directly, as well as help to activate the immune system. It is used for the treatment of cancers including multiple myeloma, chronic myeloid leukemia and hairy cell leukemia. Some patients respond better than others. A common side effect is a flulike reaction with fever, fatigue, and chills.

Lymph node removal

Lymph nodes are removed either to see whether cancerous cells are present—cells that have probably spread from a primary cancer site elsewhere—or when it is known that the nodes are cancerous and surgery is thought to be the best way to treat the malignancy.

Lymph nodes are small beanlike swellings that occur at intervals throughout the lymphatic system (see page 30). They are found in different parts of the body; in particular, there are groups of nodes in the neck and behind the ear, around the armpit, in the area of the groin, and in various locations within the abdomen.

LYMPH NODE BIOPSY

Because a lymph node biopsy involves an operation, it is usually only performed when other, simpler, tests have not been helpful. For example, swollen lymph nodes (lymphadenopathy, see page 135) can be caused by infections, and in these cases, blood tests for infectious mononucleosis or HIV may be sufficient for a diagnosis.

Fine needle aspiration

Some easily felt lymph nodes just under the skin can be biopsied using a fine needle: This is often called fine needle aspiration. A local anesthetic makes this a painless process, and a hospital stay is not necessary. However, only small samples can be obtained by fine needle aspiration.

SURGICAL LYMPH NODE REMOVAL

For a biopsy involving deeper lymph nodes, or when a large sample is required or a number of lymph nodes are removed as a cancer treatment, patients are given a general anesthetic and the lymph nodes are taken out by a surgeon. This requires a few days in the hospital.

After the operation

Often, the only adverse effect is soreness that wears off in a few weeks. Sometimes, however, the removal of lymph nodes can cause a gradual swelling of the limb or area

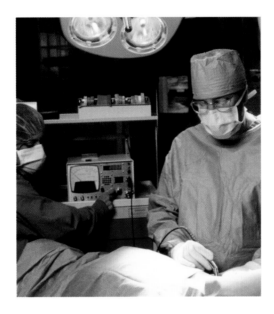

affected that is known as lymphedema. Unfortunately, this cannot be eradicated completely, but it can generally be controlled by circulation-boosting activities such as massage, exercise, and wearing compression sleeves or stockings, as appropriate.

Selective surgery
The surgeon removes only those lymph nodes in the region of the patient's breast that have been identified as cancerous by sentinel lymph node mapping.

ON THE CUTTING EDGE

Sentinel lymph node mapping

The traditional way of testing for and arresting the spread of breast cancer is to remove 15 or more lymph nodes from the area surrounding the breast; only when they are examined in a laboratory does it become known which ones (if any) contained cancer cells. Inevitably, damage to the nerves, muscle and other tissues surrounding the nodes means the patient faces a painful recovery, with stiffness, swelling, and loss of movement in the affected arm that may be permanent. Now there is a new procedure called sentinel node mapping that is much less invasive. A few hours before the operation to remove lymph nodes, a radiologist injects a solution of radioactive tracer material and blue dye into the breast, around the site of the cancer. This solution will collect in any "sentinel" lymph nodes in the area that contain cancerous cells. The surgeon then knows exactly which lymph nodes are cancerous and will take care to remove only these in the operation that follows.

Stem cell transplantation

Doctors can now take immature "stem" cells, capable of developing into several different types of mature cell, and use them to boost the bone marrow of a patient whose marrow is starting to fail. Bone marrow transplant is a type of stem cell transplant.

WHAT ARE STEM CELLS?

Stem cells are very immature cells that have the capability to develop into a wide range of mature cells. Stem cells are present in large numbers in the blood of newborn babies. They are harder to find in adults but are present in small quantities in the blood and especially in bone marrow. Stem cells from adult bone marrow have been shown to be capable of growing into mature brain cells. It is possible that in the future such cells could be used to treat patients who have severe spinal cord injuries, for example. At the moment, the main medical use of stem cells is to replace stem cells in the recipient's bone marrow that have been damaged by chemotherapy.

TAKING STEM CELLS FROM BONE MARROW

Stem cells are removed relatively easily from the bone marrow. The donor is given a general anesthetic, and several bone aspirates are taken from the pelvic bones. About one pint of bone marrow is removed—this may yield several million stem cells.

It is also possible to remove stem cells from a donor's blood. First, the donor is given a series of injections to increase the number of stem cells in the circulation. Then some blood is taken and the stem cells are extracted from it. This process is less traumatic for the donor but may yield fewer cells than bone marrow aspiration.

Conditioning the recipient's marrow

Prior to stem cell transplant, room must be made in the recipient's bone marrow. The recipient's marrow has to be destroyed by cytotoxic chemotherapy drugs in order to allow the donor stem cells to produce new marrow. This process is referred to as conditioning. In cases of cancer, lymphoma, and leukemia, these conditioning drugs will also help to eradicate cancer cells.

RECEIVING THE DONOR STEM CELLS

The donor's stem cells are infused intravenously into the recipient through a Hickman catheter inserted into a vein. It takes about a month for the new stem cells to grow and restore the blood counts to normal. During this period, the recipient is kept in isolation in the hospital because of the increased likelihood of infection and bleeding associated with a low blood cell count. Sometimes the stem cells fail to multiply— this is known as graft failure.

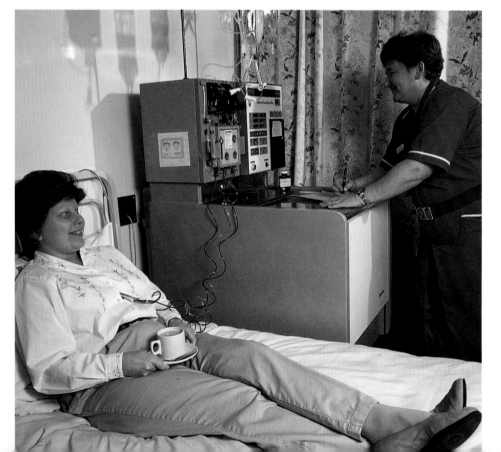

Peripheral blood stem cell (PBSC) donation
First the prospective PBSC donor is given an injection of natural growth factors to stimulate her bone marrow to produce extra PBSC. Then, as shown here, the donor's blood is run through a separating machine that removes the PBSCs, which will be given to a patient in need of PBSC transplantation.

WHEN A STEM CELL TRANSPLANT IS NEEDED

- In babies with severe genetic problems affecting the cells of the bone marrow, such as babies with severe combined immunodeficiency (SCID) or thalassemia.
- In cancers of the blood cells (leukemia, lymphoma, and myeloma), a stem cell transplant replaces bone marrow damaged by chemotherapy undertaken to reduce the number of cancerous cells made in the marrow. In some cases, initial chemotherapy reduces the number of malignant cells to almost zero. When some cancer cells remain, it may be possible to give stronger chemotherapy that will hopefully eradicate the cancer cells. But stronger chemotherapy almost always damages normal bone marrow cells, and then a stem cell transplant is required to replace the damaged marrow.
- In cases of bone marrow failure, a stem cell transplant may be used if other measures are not working. For example, when a patient has developed bone marrow failure (see page 139) after taking a particular drug, the drug is stopped and the patient is observed to see if the marrow will recover without extra help. If this does not happen, stem cell transplantation may be carried out.
- In some cases of severe autoimmune disease, the patient's immune system continues to attack normal tissues even after strong immunosuppressive drugs have been given. More potent immunosuppressive drugs may control the autoimmune disease but will also destroy the immune system and healthy bone marrow, making stem cell transplantation necessary.

ON THE CUTTINH EDGE

Stem cells from "cord blood"

Recently, cord blood has been used as a source of stem cells. Cord blood is the blood left in the umbilical cord after it has been cut off a newborn baby. Normally it is thrown away. There is only about a quarter of a pint of blood in the umbilical cord and not many stem cells are present; however, the cells seem to be particularly good at regenerating a recipient's bone marrow, and there may be a reduced risk of graft versus host disease, one of the most serious complications of stem cell transplant (see page 122). Cord blood can be frozen for several months. In the future, cord blood may be stored in special banks so that the stem cells can subsequently be used for anyone that needs them. Shown here is a test sample being taken from a bag of cord blood before a transfusion.

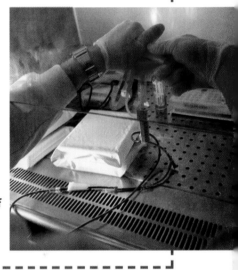

❝ DONATING BONE MARROW

When I registered as a potential bone marrow donor, the bone marrow registry took a blood sample to identify my HLA type, and the information was entered on the registry computer.

Three years later, the registry contacted me: They had a potential recipient for my bone marrow. I went to see them for more blood tests and a full medical exam, and, these having *proven OK, a date was set for the donation. I checked into the hospital the night before the operation. The procedure itself took about an hour and was performed under general anesthetic.*

The surgeon had explained how he would use a hollow needle and syringe to extract about a pint of marrow from my pelvic bones. When I came around, I felt very tired and also very sore around *my lower back. I spent the following night in the hospital recovering. The doctor told me it would take 4–6 weeks for my bone marrow to replenish itself. It was a few weeks before the soreness disappeared entirely, too.*

Nevertheless, I feel happy that I was able to give the person who received my bone marrow a chance of recovery from his or her illness.

❞

AUTOLOGOUS STEM CELL TRANSPLANT

The simplest form of stem cell transplant involves using the patient's own marrow. It is particularly appropriate for patients with leukemia when there is a high risk of cancer returning after moderate doses of chemotherapy. A quantity of bone marrow is removed from the patient, who then receives a high dose of chemotherapy, which destroys cancer cells and normal bone marrow cells. While this is happening, all cancer cells are removed from the extracted bone marrow sample. The "cleaned up" marrow is then returned to the patient. This technique is relatively straightforward because there are no genetic differences between the marrow and the recipient.

THE CHANCES OF REJECTION

In some ways, stem cell transplant is like any other transplant: If there are genetic differences between donor and recipient, the transplant will be rejected. The potential for these differences is mainly in the HLA (human leukocyte antigen) genes: If donor and recipient have different tissue types, the recipient will reject the stem cell transplant. The same rules therefore apply to stem cell transplant as to any other transplant: Transplants between identical twins will work well; transplants between siblings have a one in four chance of working well—when the HLA types happen to be identical. The chances of a random donor having the same tissue type and the transplant working well are very small.

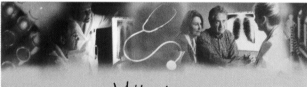

Milestones
IN MEDICINE

Stem cell research on embryos is controversial in the United States because of the complex moral and ethical issues surrounding the embryos. In 2002, the U.S. government announced that it would fund research on already-existing chains of stem cells (they replicate) but not on new stem cells.

Graft versus host disease

Stem cell transplants differ from other transplants in that the immune cells will grow out of the donor stem cells. If there are genetic differences between the donor and the recipient, the new immune cells, derived from the donor, will attack tissues throughout the recipient's body. This is called graft versus host disease. Acute graft versus host disease happens very soon after the transplant and attacks numerous tissues throughout the body. Chronic graft versus host disease usually causes skin and lung problems several months after transplantation.

The risk of graft versus host disease is reduced by ensuring that donor and recipient have identical HLA (tissue) types, if possible. However, other genetic differences between the donor and recipient are likely and cannot be predicted by tissue typing technologies. Most stem cell transplant patients therefore take immunosuppressive drugs to reduce the risk as much as possible.

Registering as a potential unrelated donor

The chances of someone who needs a stem cell transplant having an identical twin are very slim. The chances of having a sibling who can act as a donor are also low. As a result, unrelated donors are increasingly being used for transplants. However, unrelated donor stem cell transplant only works if there is an exact HLA match. Therefore, the more people that register their HLA type with a stem cell registry, the more likely it is that someone in need of a stem cell transplant will find a successful match.

Donors need to be healthy and 18 to 40 years old. If a patient requires a transplant of a particular donor's HLA type, the donor is contacted and a blood sample is taken for a cross-match to confirm that the risk of stem cell rejection or graft versus host disease is as low as possible. All being well, the donor's bone marrow is then removed and transplanted into the recipient.

Banks for cord blood too

In the future, banks of cord blood may be used as a resource for children who need stem cell transplantation. Stem cells from cord blood are much less likely to cause graft versus host disease but are only available in small amounts and so are not usually suitable for adult patients.

Stem cell gene therapy for SCID

Every year, a handful of boys are born with X-linked severe combined immunodeficiency (SCID). This condition makes them unable to fight infections of any kind. Stem cell gene therapy can transform their life prospects.

WHAT IS X-LINKED SCID?

In X-linked severe combined immunodeficiency (SCID), there is a mutation, an incorrect DNA sequence, in the gene that codes for a protein—the common gamma (gc) chain. Without the gc chain, there are no T cells and no natural killer (NK) cells, both vital for fighting invading microorganisms. This means that babies born with X-linked SCID succumb to even the mildest infections. Untreated, they die of infections within the first year of life.

Even though B cells develop, because the young patients lack the T cells that normally help B cells function properly, the B cells do not produce enough useful antibodies, further impairing the immune response.

LIFE IN A "BUBBLE"

Standard treatment for children with SCID consists of lifelong injections of immunoglobulin (antibodies from donor blood) and stem cell transplantation, if a tissue-matched donor can be found. To protect the patients from infection, they may at certain stages have to live in a sterile room—a so-called "bubble" with filtered, cleansed air—and be given daily antibiotics. Parents must wear sterile gowns and face masks and can have only minimal contact with their sick child.

THE NEW TREATMENT

The first step in the new stem cell gene therapy—developed by doctors in France and the UK—is to remove some of the child's bone marrow cells from the hip bone using a needle and syringe and under general anesthetic.

In an incubator and under sterile conditions, these bone marrow cells are mixed in a kind of plastic bag with growth factors that selectively stimulate the stem cells. A virus that carries the correct human form of the gc chain gene is added to these defective stem cells. The virus itself causes no harm but delivers a normal gc chain gene to the stem cell nucleus, where it can take over from the defective gene and rescue the vital immune cell function. The process of selecting the cells and putting them in contact with the virus takes about three days, after which

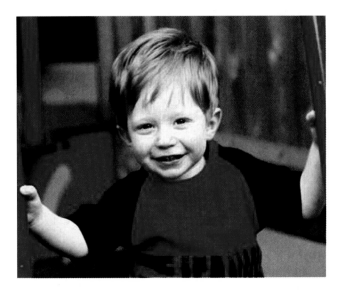

Ready to live a normal life for the first time
Rhys Evans from South Wales was one of the first children to have received stem cell gene therapy for SCID. He left London's Great Ormond Street Hospital in 2002 with the hope that he will be able to enjoy a normal childhood from now on.

about 20 million cells are put back into the patient by injection in a process that resembles a blood transfusion.

In most other transplant procedures, the recipient's bone marrow must be emptied out to make room for donor cells; this is usually done by killing the recipient's cells by irradiation. The therapy being pioneered for X-linked SCID is quite different: Bone marrow cells are already so sparse that there is no need to "prepare" a patient to accommodate the corrected cells.

After receiving their modified stem cells, patients slowly acquire immune cells. T cells are usually detected in the blood four to six months after a stem cell transplant but appear two to four months after stem cell gene therapy and are about three times as abundant. It has now been several years since the first young patients with X-linked SCID received stem cell gene therapy. So far, it appears that their immune systems have been successfully repaired. In the future, gene therapy may be adapted for other diseases caused by mutations, such as hemophilia.

Fighting childhood leukemia

The outlook for children with leukemia has never been better. Although it is often in children that leukemia progresses most rapidly, more children than ever before now go into remission with the prospect of a healthy adult life.

The types of leukemia to which children are most likely to fall victim are acute lymphoblastic leukemia or acute myeloid leukemia—usually aggressive, fast-growing tumors—or chronic myeloid leukemia, which begins slowly but can transform into a much more aggressive disease.

In children, the first signs are often loss of energy, tiredness, and fever. There may be persistent infections, nosebleeds, bruising, and aching joints or bones. The disease is usually diagnosed via a blood test and bone marrow biopsy.

Every year, about 2200 children are diagnosed with leukemia in the U.S. Of these, about three-quarters are cured (a remission of five years after treatment is generally considered as a cure). The reasons that medicine is now enjoying higher success rates against leukemia in children are early diagnosis and more sophisticated treatment programs. The principal weapons in medicine's fight against this disease are chemotherapy, radiation, and stem cell transplant.

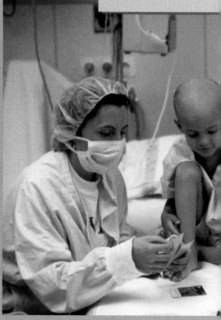

A boy receiving chemotherapy for leukemia plays cards with his mother.

Leukemic blood cells

A colored scanning electron micrograph (SEM) of the blood of a patient with leukemia shows a typical overabundance of white blood cells. They form a marked contrast with the SEM of healthy blood shown below. The term "leukemia" covers any of a group of cancerous diseases in which the overproduction of immature, abnormal white blood cells suppresses the production of red blood cells, platelets, and normal white blood cells. This leads to a vastly increased susceptibility to infection, plus anemia and problems caused by the blood not clotting properly. If leukemia is not adequately treated, it will ultimately prove fatal.

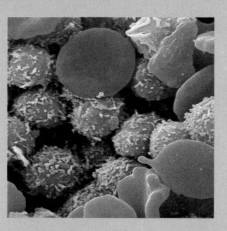

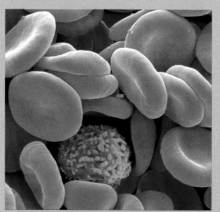

Treatment options

How each case of leukemia is treated varies from child to child, depending on factors such as the precise type of leukemia, how aggressive it is, and the success of any previous treatments.

CHEMOTHERAPY

With acute lymphoblastic leukemia, chemotherapy treatment is started as soon as possible after diagnosis. This involves the injection into a vein of a cytotoxic (cell-poisoning) drug that will kill cancerous cells—but also some healthy cells. If the leukemia returns, chemotherapy is given again, sometimes at a higher dosage.

RADIATION

Radiation may be used to kill any leukemia calls that have spread into the fluid around the brain and spinal cord. It is sometimes given after chemotherapy to "mop up" any cancer cells still remaining in this cerebrospinal fluid.

STEM CELL TRANSPLANTATION

When chemotherapy treatment destroys so many healthy cells in the bone marrow that the child's immune system has been severely damaged, stem cell transplantation (see page 120) is the treatment of choice to rejuvenate the immune system.

ISOLATION

Both chemotherapy (possibly coupled with radiation) and stem cell transplantation can affect the immune system so badly that any infection can pose a danger to the patient. In these circumstances, the best protection for the patient is isolation in a sterile room within the hospital.

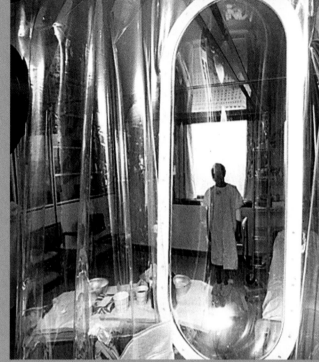

A pediatric leukemia patient in a sterile isolation room in a hospital following chemotherapy and stem cell transplantation. The few people allowed into the room have to "scrub down" and put on special clothing before entering.

A happy outcome

Joanne Mills—shown here, second from the left, standing next to consultant oncologist Dr. Alison Leiper—was diagnosed with acute lymphoblastic leukemia at the age of nine. Acute lymphoblastic leukemia is the most common of all the cancers contracted by children. Joanne clearly remembers being whisked into London's Great Ormond Street Hospital for Children, where treatment was started immediately. The outcome was successful and she has been leukemia-free ever since.

In the not-so-distant past, some treatments for leukemia could make it difficult for some patients to go on to have children in later life, but happily the situation is now much improved. Joanne is pictured here with her daughter and son.

Great Ormond Street Hospital for Children, founded in 1852, is the largest care center in Great Britain for children with leukemia and one of the world's leading research centers in the field of child health. In 2002, Great Ormond Street Hospital and 21 other specialized pediatric oncology centers included within the UK Children's Cancer Study Group celebrated 25 years of increasing success in fighting

childhood cancer. The number of children who develop cancer each year in the UK—approximately one in every 600 age 15 or under—has remained constant for the last 25 years and longer, but cure rates for some cancers have almost doubled in that time, going from four out of ten to nearly eight out of ten.

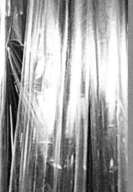

Organ transplants and immunosuppression

The transplant revolution is relatively recent. The reason is that although the surgical techniques for transplanting organs have in some cases been known for some time, immunosuppression therapy that prevents organs being rejected has only gotten off the ground in the last 30 years or so.

Transplantation is the treatment of choice for patients with end-stage organ failure. Solid organs that may be transplanted include the kidney, the heart, liver, lungs, the pancreas, and small intestine. The reason that kidney transplants are the most commonly performed is because living people (usually relatives) can donate one of their two healthy kidneys. In addition, patients with kidney failure can be kept alive on dialysis machines until an organ is available. Patients with severe heart, lung, or liver failure are not so fortunate and need a transplant urgently.

HOW DEMAND OUTSTRIPS SUPPLY

From January to December 2002 in the United States, 25,765 transplants were performed (double-organ transplants count as one) with organs from 12,794 donors. There were still 80,769 people waiting for transplants.

Most organs are from brainstem-dead cadaver donors. There are never enough cadaver donors, however—and the number is declining because of a decrease in how many people are killed in road accidents and by intracranial bleeding.

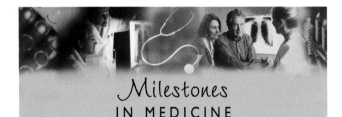

Milestones
IN MEDICINE

1954 First successful kidney transplant, between identical twins in Boston.
1963 Thomas Starzl carries out the first successful liver transplant, in Denver.
1967 In Cape Town, South Africa, Christiaan Barnard performs the first successful heart transplant.
1967 First successful pancreas transplant.
1984 First heart–liver transplant is performed, again by Thomas Starzl, in Pittsburgh.
1990 First successful heart–lung transplant is performed.
1991 First successful small intestine transplant.

Increasing numbers of living kidney donors

Transplant numbers have been kept constant by an increase in the number of living donors. There were 6232 living donor kidney transplants in the United States in 2002, compared with 2494 in 1992. This is more than 40 percent of all kidney transplants in 2002.

Live related donation can be very safe because a related donor is genetically similar or even identical to the recipient. It is also possible for an unrelated living donor to donate a kidney. This is less likely to be successful because of genetic differences and could possibly lead to organ selling, which is of course illegal in the U.S.

MATCHING DONOR AND RECIPIENT

If a transplant is to be a success, it is essential that the donated organ is transplanted into a recipient with a compatible blood type. If not, the transplanted organ will be rejected. In addition, there is also a procedure called tissue typing, or matching, which examines the HLA profile of donor and recipient tissues to assess compatibility of their antigens.

There are protein chains called human leukocyte antigens (HLA) in almost every cell in the body. Everyone has a particular HLA type, known as the tissue type, inherited from the parents. We each have two HLA A antigens, two HLA B antigens, and two HLA DR antigens; these are made up of one A, one B, and one DR passed down from each parent. The function of HLA is to regulate the immune response. It plays a key role in enabling the body to distinguish self from non-self.

What is the importance of a close tissue match?

HLA matching is important in heart transplantation, but sometimes there is not enough time to perform a cross-match (a compatibility test). Many studies have shown there is no need to HLA-match liver grafts.

With kidneys, however, the closer the HLA match between kidney donor organ and recipient, the greater the chance of a transplant being accepted by the recipient's body. There is a 25 percent chance of two siblings sharing the same tissue type, a 50 percent chance of siblings being a half match, and a 25 percent chance of siblings being totally mismatched. Parents are a half match for their children, and children are a half match for their parents. There is only a small chance of an unrelated donor–recipient pair having a good HLA match.

WHY A LIVING DONOR IS PREFERABLE

- It takes less time to transplant an organ from donor to recipient—a matter of a few hours at most. This is because the operation can be planned well in advance, so that the pretransplant tests that delay a cadaver donor transplant can be carried out in the days before the organ is taken from the live donor. The longer a kidney, for example, is kept on ice, the less likely it is that it will work at once. Immediate functioning is a major factor in successful organ transplant outcome.
- A living donor is given a thorough checkup, something that is not possible with a cadaver donor.
- If a living donor is already lined up, a patient in need of a new kidney is more likely to receive a transplant before having to begin dialysis, which increases the chances of the transplant being a success.

DONATION AFTER THE DONOR'S DEATH

Usually, a cadaver donor has sustained irreversible brainstem death and subsequently been maintained on a ventilator machine. There are also "non-heart-beating"

More than half of the U.S. population has signed a donor card.

donors who have not been given assisted ventilation (a machine has not been keeping them breathing); these are very rare at present.

Before the operation

Three conditions have to be met before cadaver donation can take place.

- As is the case for blood donors, the donor must not have infections such as hepatitis or HIV and must not have a life-threatening condition such as cancer.
- Very careful testing must confirm irreversible brainstem death (see page 128).
- There must be consent from the donor's family.

As soon as a family grants permission for a patient's organs to be used, the transplant coordinator communicates with intensive care staff, operating room staff, and transplant teams to arrange a time for the donation, and blood is sent to a transplant laboratory to determine the patient's tissue type.

Harvesting the organs

As many as 50 people can receive organs or tissue from a donor. Just before the operation begins, the cadaver donor is taken off the ventilator (if applicable). First the cardiac team retrieves the heart and lungs. It is important that these organs are transplanted within 12 hours of removal from the donor. The liver is removed next; this should be transplanted as soon as possible. Then the kidneys and pancreas are taken out.

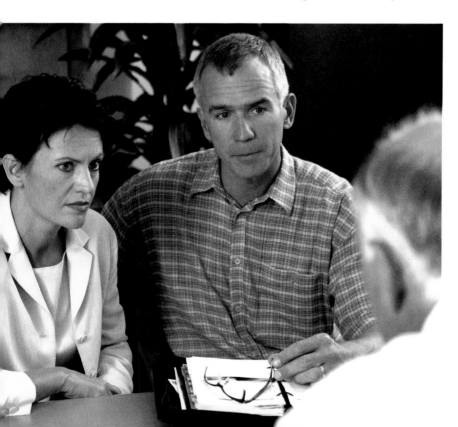

Seeking permission from relatives
In the U.S., relatives of someone who has just died and is a potential organ donor are always asked to consent to the donation of organs, whether or not the potential donor carried a donor card or joined a donor register. If the family of the donor refuses consent, the donation does not take place.

IMMUNOSUPPRESSIVE THERAPY

The body's immune system naturally recognizes transplanted organs as foreign and rejects them. For this reason, immunosuppression—interrupting this normal tendency—plays a major role in the success of any organ transplant.

The immunosuppressive regimen has two critical phases: first the immediate postimplant phase, when it is necessary to prevent sensitization of mature recipient cells capable of recognizing the newly transplanted organ, and then cumulative unresponsiveness to the new organ, which develops as the recipient is continually exposed to donor HLA from the organ.

Currently, there does not seem to be one best immunosuppressive regimen suitable for all patients. As doctors learn more about individual immune responses, it becomes possible to tailor specific immunosuppressive regimens to the needs of the individual patient. All the drugs listed below are still in use—in most cases, patients are treated with a combination of two or three. One trend is that fewer steroids are being prescribed as more potent drugs become available.

Steroids and azathioprine

When transplantation surgery began to take off in the 1970s, the immunosuppression regime was limited to steroids and azathioprine. Steroids have a nonspecific immunosuppressive effect, acting by damping down the inflammatory response. Azathioprine interferes with the metabolism of cells involved in the immune response, and stops them from proliferating.

Cyclosporin (CSA)

Cyclosporin (CSA) arrived on the scene in the early 1980s, and from the mid-1980s to mid-1990s—the "cyclosporin era"—a great improvement was seen in graft survival figures. CSA acts by inhibiting the production of chemical signals that act between cells, thus preventing cells from proliferating. The earliest form of CSA was replaced in the late 90s by a more effective form marketed as Neoral, which has been shown to provide better overall immunosuppression. One drawback with CSA, however, is that in high doses the drug damages the kidneys—as shown by heart transplant patients who have gone into renal failure as a result of CSA treatment. CSA can also cause the gums to grow over the teeth (gum hypertrophy) and excessive hair growth (hypertrichosis).

How can we be sure a potential donor is really dead?

TALKING POINT

A common worry is whether a potential donor whose heartbeat and breathing have been maintained on a ventilator is actually dead. Any patient on life support who is identified as a potential donor must undergo a series of tests at two different times by a medical team other than the transplant team. Only if the patient is completely unresponsive in both sets of tests can the patient be diagnosed as brain dead.

Other immunosuppressive drugs

- Tacrolimus (FK506, Prograf) is derived from a fungus, like CSA, and has a similar mode of action, though it acts on a wider range of chemical signals. It too is nephrotoxic (damages the kidneys), but it doesn't cause gum hypertrophy or hypertrichosis. When it was first introduced, there was concern over the high incidence of diabetes caused, but with more widespread use and a better understanding of therapeutic blood levels, this has lessened. There is evidence that tacrolimus may be a better immunosuppressive agent than CSA after a liver transplant. Patients with severe CSA side effects can benefit from a switch to tacrolimus, and the drug is used as a "rescue agent" when patients have rejection episodes not treatable by an increase in steroids.

- Sirolimus (Rapamycin) works by competing with the action of chemical signals on target cells and can be used in conjunction with CSA. Sirolimus works synergistically with CSA. Though sirolimus is not harmful to kidneys, it does cause high cholesterol levels. A large proportion of patients involved in sirolimus trials have had to be treated with lipid-lowering drugs.

- Mycophenolate mofetil (MMF, CellCept) inhibits chemical signalling by interfering with cell metabolism. UK trials showed a 50 percent reduction in acute rejection when MMF was used in conjunction with CSA, and in the U.S., MMF has virtually replaced azathioprine in clinical practice. Use of the drug in the UK has been restricted by cost, but it is now effectively used in conjunction with steroids in patients with chronic CSA nephrotoxicity and is considered to be of significant benefit in pancreas transplants.

• A monoclonal antibody (anti-CD3, OKT3) or a polyclonal antibody (anti-lymphocyte globulin, ALG, or anti-thymocyte globulin, ATG) is used to help patients experiencing a rejection crisis. These agents deplete the cells responsible for rejection so the transplanted organ is not attacked. It's important that sufficient cells remain to guard against infection so that a balance between preventing rejection and preventing infection is reached.

SUCCESSFUL TRANSPLANTATION

Various factors influence whether a transplant will be successful and enable a return to a normal lifestyle. Donor factors that tip the balance in favor of a successful outcome include
• normal anatomy of the donor organ;
• evidence that the organ was working well before donation;
• the donor's age—5 to 50 years old.
Donor factors that might lead to early failure of the transplant include
• a lapse of time greater than 45 minutes from the point at which the donor's blood ceased to flow through an organ to the moment when the organ is perfused with solution and packed in ice—known as the "warm ischemia time";

• a period of more than 24 hours from the time when the organ is first perfused and chilled to the moment when the recipient's blood begins to circulate within it—the cold ischemia time; and
• evidence of infection.
Recipient factors are just as important. Factors in favor of a successful outcome are
• good HLA matching with the donor—especially HLA DR;
• lack of side effects from the immunosuppressants; and
• compliance in taking antirejection drugs, maybe for life.
Recipient factors leading to early failure include
• a previous transplant history and the formation of HLA specific antibodies;
• recurrent disease in the new organ; and
• anatomical abnormalities that make links between the donor and the recipient's blood vessels difficult.
Transplant recipients can return to a near normal life, a fact best exemplified by the Transplant Games. Quality of life should continue to improve for these patients as better immunosuppressants are developed and coupled with immunosuppressant regimens tailored to the individual needs of each recipient, and as understanding of the processes involved in rejection increases.

Transplant Games
The U.S. Transplant Games take place biannually as a four-day athletic event and a celebration of how successful a treatment organ transplantation can be. The World Transplant Games are also held every two years.

Life on immunosuppressants

Immunosuppressant drugs are taken before and after organ and tissue transplants to prevent rejection. They do so by impairing the body's ability to fight infection. How does this impact everyday life for recipients, who often have to take these drugs for the rest of their lives?

Every patient's situation is slightly different, but in general, someone on immunosuppressants can live a life as normal as anyone else's, as long as certain basic precautions and commonsense procedures are followed.

All immunosuppressant drugs increase the risk of catching an infection and of an infection doing greater harm to the body than if these drugs were not being taken. This is because these drugs impair the body's ability to recognize and respond to infection. In particular, immunosuppressants such as mycophenolate, azathioprine, and sirolimus tend to suppress white blood cells, which normally help fight infection. For this reason, doctors regularly monitor the white blood cell counts of patients on these drugs.

TIPS FOR AVOIDING INFECTIONS

There are various measures that can be taken to reduce the chances of catching an infection.

- **High hygiene standards** Practice good hand hygiene: Wash hands frequently, avoid close contact with other people who may be carrying an infection, and use gloves and a mask if having to handle pet waste.
- **Keeping the doctor informed** Report any contact with infectious illness to the doctor, so that the appropriate preventative treatment can be prescribed. Typical examples include chicken pox and the herpes virus.
- **Vaccinations before vacationing abroad** Consult the doctor about which vaccines can and cannot be taken: For example, live vaccines (that is, measles/mumps/rubella, the oral polio vaccine, and yellow fever vaccines) should not be given to a transplant recipient.
- **Going to the dentist** Check with the transplant doctor and dentist before any dental procedures are performed to find out whether or not antibiotics are needed.
- **Food poisoning** Beware of food poisoning if you are on immunosuppressants, because food poisoning can have a more dangerous effect than it would otherwise. In particular, avoid any egg and cheese products that have not been completely cooked.

DEALING WITH AN INFECTION

Early detection of an infection is crucial to avoid complications. A doctor should be notified of any signs of infection such as a sore throat, a cough, swollen lymph nodes, or mouth sores, so that the appropriate investigations and treatments can be started as soon as possible. Anyone on immunosuppressants should get immediate medical advice after an animal or insect bite or after receiving a cut or wound of any kind.

The importance of exercise
Regular exercise will help keep you healthy and ready to fight off infection. Low impact, repetitive exercises such as walking and skipping are particularly good for the bones and are a simple way to help keep the potential immunosuppressant side effect of osteoporosis at bay.

HOW TO KEEP SIDE EFFECTS TO A MINIMUM

The frequency and seriousness of the side effects of immunosuppressants are related to each drug's specific effect and the size of the dose. Some signs and symptoms can be seen or felt, but others are detected only by medical tests, so regular monitoring by a health professional is essential. The potential side effects of immunosuppressive drugs differ and will include only a few of the signs and symptoms referred to here.

- **Keep bones strong** The risk of osteoporosis can be minimized by taking vitamin D and calcium supplements as medically prescribed, by adopting a diet with enough calcium and vitamin D, by cutting down or quitting smoking and alcohol, and by doing gentle weight-bearing exercises.

- **Avoid high blood pressure** Reduce or eliminate risk factors such as high cholesterol, high salt intake, smoking, and obesity. A diet high in fruit and vegetables and low in salt, sugar, and fat is best. Take blood pressure medicines precisely as directed by the doctor.

- **Minimize swelling** A mild accumulation of fluid in the body can often be alleviated by a few commonsense measures, such as drinking lots of water to encourage fluid to pass through the body; reducing salt intake; increasing physical activity; avoiding tight clothes, jewelry, and shoes; and elevating the feet whenever possible—by raising the foot of the bed, for example.

- **Bruising** Bruising can be avoided by careful blood monitoring by the doctor. Patients should report bruising in unusual areas such as the chest, inner thighs, or inner arms immediately.

- **Avoid high lipid (fat) levels (hyperlipidemia)** The presence of an abnormally high concentration of fats in the blood often occurs with immunosuppressant use, and it increases the risk of heart disease. The doctor can help by keeping a regular check on blood lipid levels and by prescribing medicines called "statins" to control cholesterol levels. Patients can help by exercising regularly and adopting a low-fat, low-cholesterol diet.

- **Tremors** Report any tremors to the doctor immediately so the cause can be identified and the right treatment set in place. Simple stretching exercises are sometimes enough to temporarily relieve the problem.

- **Conquer headaches** Acetaminophen is safe for transplant patients to take. By contrast, ibuprofen (Advil) and naproxen (Naprosyn) can suppress kidney function and should be avoided by transplant recipients. Report any severe or persistent headaches to the doctor immediately.

- **Maintain hair condition** Hair can be weakened and may even break off at the roots. Help hair stay healthy by avoiding perming or dyeing, and covering it when sunbathing or swimming.

- **Skin care** Wear sunscreen and protective clothing in the sun. Notify the doctor at once if any moles change in any way.

- **Gums** Careful attention to dental hygiene is the way to help avoid overgrown or bleeding gums.

Removing the spleen

An operation to remove the spleen is called a splenectomy. This is sometimes performed on people who have a severely enlarged spleen (splenomegaly). More often, however, the spleen is removed because it has been ruptured in an accident.

The spleen has two major roles in controlling infection.
- It acts as a filter to remove bacteria from the blood.
- It contains special B cells that make antibodies against bacteria, for example against pneumococcus, which can cause serious infections including pneumonia.

A lot of blood flows through the spleen, and if the spleen is even slightly damaged following physical injury, there can be massive internal bleeding. In such an emergency, a surgeon may decide it is better to remove the spleen rather than attempt to repair it.

The operation

A surgeon may opt to remove a spleen by traditional surgical methods or by using the newer techniques of laparoscopic or "keyhole" surgery. Before the operation begins, tests will have been carried out to find out as much as possible about the spleen's condition—the extent of any trauma or enlargement in particular. The patient is given antibiotics just before the operation to cut down on the risk of infection.

After the operation

Patients can manage quite well without a spleen, but they are left more prone to infection than before. The risk of sepsis from bacterial infection is greatest among children, so a splenectomy should be avoided if at all possible if the patient is a child.

Splenectomy patients can develop severe septicemia after even trivial infections, such as a splinter in the finger: Patients can become severely ill in just a few minutes. For this reason, all splenectomy patients should wear an alert bracelet or tag. Even more important, patients who have had a splenectomy should take simple antibiotics such as penicillin daily. In the U.S., patients are advised to take penicillin for the first few years after the operation; in the U.K., splenectomy patients are often advised to take penicillin for the rest of their lives. Additionally, splenectomy patients need to be vaccinated against pneumococcus and meningococcus (which can cause septicemia) in order to encourage the immune system to make antibodies.

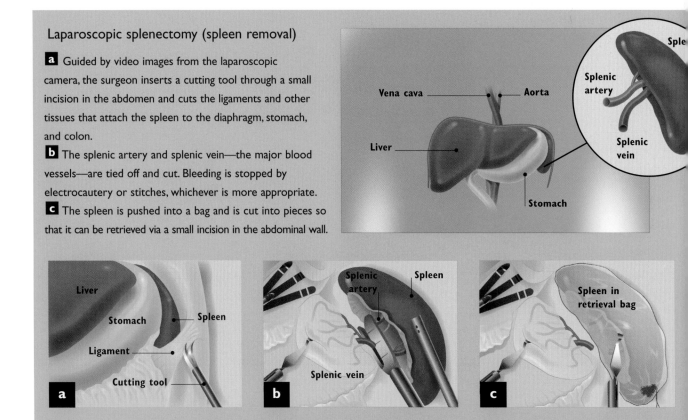

Laparoscopic splenectomy (spleen removal)

a Guided by video images from the laparoscopic camera, the surgeon inserts a cutting tool through a small incision in the abdomen and cuts the ligaments and other tissues that attach the spleen to the diaphragm, stomach, and colon.

b The splenic artery and splenic vein—the major blood vessels—are tied off and cut. Bleeding is stopped by electrocautery or stitches, whichever is more appropriate.

c The spleen is pushed into a bag and is cut into pieces so that it can be retrieved via a small incision in the abdominal wall.

Vena cava — Aorta — Sple — Splenic artery — Liver — Splenic vein — Stomach

Liver — Stomach — Spleen — Ligament — Cutting tool

Splenic artery — Spleen — Splenic vein

Spleen in retrieval bag

A to Z

OF DISEASES AND DISORDERS

This section gives information on the main illnesses and medical conditions that affect the blood and immune system.

This index is divided into two sections: Symptoms, and Diseases and disorders. Within these divisions, entries are arranged alphabetically, and each is structured in a similar way:

What are the causes?

What are the symptoms?

How is it diagnosed?

What are the treatment options?

SYMPTOMS

ANEMIA
A reduction in the amount of oxygen-rich hemoglobin in the blood.

Hemoglobin in the blood gives a healthy color to the skin. Sometimes anemia is suggested by a pale appearance, but many white people have naturally pale complexions. The mucous membranes of the mouth and the whites of the eyes are therefore better places to look for the pallor of anemia.

What are the causes?
Anemia can be caused by an iron or vitamin deficiency, blood loss, or chronic illness. It can also be genetic in origin or a side effect of certain medications.

How is it diagnosed?
The most common symptom is fatigue regardless of how much sleep and rest the patient is getting. If the anemia is more severe, the patient may feel his or her heart beating inside the chest (palpitations) or have shortness of breath. It is important to remember, however, that these symptoms can also be caused by other medical problems.

   The doctor will examine the patient and take account of the symptoms. A complete blood count (p. 105) will then be taken to confirm the anemia; this may also give clues to the cause of the anemia.

What are the treatment options?
The type of treatment will depend on the underlying cause of the anemia and therefore varies greatly from case to case (p. 114).

BLEEDING
Any excessive bleeding warrants getting medical advice.

What are the causes?
Excessive bleeding can occur if there are problems in the relevant organ. For example, heavy periods can indicate a hormonal imbalance or the presence of fibroids. Nosebleeds can indicate infections in the nose, or a problem with the blood-clotting system. Bleeding can also occur in people who have been prescribed too many anticoagulants such as warfarin.

How is it diagnosed?
In the case of a problem with the blood-clotting system, there may be bleeding from several sites, for example from the gums as well as the nose. In other instances, the bleeding may not be immediately obvious: In the eye, it can impair vision, and bleeding into joints causes pain and swelling. These symptoms could mean that either the platelets (as in immune thrombocytopenia) or the clotting proteins (as in hemophilia) are not working.

What are the treatment options?
First, the bleeding must be stopped. Taking iron tablets is usually sufficient to replace red blood cells lost because of bleeding, but in the most severe cases, a blood transfusion may be needed.

BRUISING
Bruises are areas of bleeding into the skin and are perfectly normal after bumps and injury to the skin.

What are the causes?
Most healthy children get bruises from time to time from heavy duty playing. In the elderly, bruising can occur because of the looseness of the tissues under the skin.

   Excessive bruises can occur when there is no clear-cut history of trauma. They can sometimes happen because of infections, such as meningococcal meningitis, so if a child or teenager (those most commonly affected by this disease) develops small bruises on the skin, fever, and headache, it is important to get immediate medical advice. Abnormal bruises also occur when the clotting system is not working (see Bleeding).

What are the treatment options?
Elevation and an ice pack may help in cases in which the cause is a trauma. Arnica cream is reputed to lessen the severity of bruises if applied immediately after a trauma. Otherwise, treatment depends on the cause of the bruising.

FEVER
This means raised temperature and is usually associated with specific diseases.

Normal temperature for most people is 98.6°F, although some people have a normal temperature about 1°F higher.

What are the causes?

Fever usually indicates infection, and it develops as the body's immune system attempts to fight the infection. In children, temperature can rise rapidly; in adults, it may not rise as much but can cause more discomfort.

How is it diagnosed?

Raised temperature and feeling hot are the most common symptoms. Feverish people are often sweaty and have shivering attacks. Fever may cause seizures in children.

Fever should be confirmed by taking the patient's temperature with a thermometer. The infectious cause of fever is often obvious, such as with a sore throat or cough with sputum production, for example. Sometimes, however, the cause is not immediately obvious, and in these cases, blood and urine tests and perhaps X-rays may be required. Occasionally, a fever can be an early symptom of lymphoma or cancer.

What are the treatment options?

Treatment depends on the cause of the fever, but drinking plenty of fluids and taking aspirin or another analgesic will usually be the first treatment advised. If the cause is a specific disease, such as measles, treatment will be appropriate for the disease.

LYMPHADENOPATHY

Swelling of the lymph nodes, or glands, which are scattered through the body.

Lymph node swelling is an important clinical sign that always needs to be investigated, especially if it has persisted over several weeks (that is, if it has become chronic). The lymph nodes are very close to the surface in the neck, armpits, and groin and can easily be felt when enlarged. Deeper lymph nodes are found in the chest and abdomen; enlargement of these nodes may be detected by X-ray or scanning techniques.

What are the causes?

Lymph nodes may be swollen in four different situations.

- **Acute infection** Lymph nodes are the manufacturing site for lymphocytes, the white cells that form a crucial part of the immune system. When an infection occurs, for example a sore throat caused by a viral infection, the local lymph nodes swell up. This happens because white cells take small samples of the virus to the lymph nodes in the locality to stimulate lymphocytes. Lymphocytes that recognize the specific virus will respond by dividing to produce many more virus-specific lymphocytes. The process is organized by specialized lymphocytes known as helper cells (CD4 cells). The new lymphocytes created in the process may produce antibodies (B cells) that will help kill the infection. Other specialized lymphocytes (cytotoxic cells) also help kill viruses. In the case of a viral sore throat, lymph nodes in the neck swell up because of all the new cells produced.

  In these situations, there may be an increase in the number of lymphocytes in the blood, because the immune system throughout the body becomes activated. The immune system is capable of dealing with most infections very quickly, and the lymph node swelling usually settles after a few days making further investigation unnecessary.

- **Chronic infection** Some infections are not easily cleared by the immune system. For example, the bacteria that cause tuberculosis evade the antibodies and cytotoxic cells produced by the immune system. HIV infection also cannot easily be cleared. In both these situations, lymph node swelling will persist for weeks or months. In the case of HIV infection, an HIV test will produce a diagnosis. In the case of tuberculosis, biopsy of the lymph nodes may be the only way of confirming the cause of the problem.

- **Cancer** The immune system's response to cancer can be a bit like its response to infection. White cells take samples of the cancerous cells to the local lymph nodes and the immune system tries to find cells that are capable of killing them. In breast cancer, for example, this results in the lymph nodes in the armpits swelling as they try to respond to the cancer. In this case, a lump in the breast is usually present, and both the lump and the lymph nodes are removed through surgery.

  In other cases, for example with throat cancer, the primary cancer may be hard to detect, and chronically swollen lymph nodes in the neck may be the first sign. Doctors can diagnose throat cancer by doing a biopsy on the swollen nodes, as well as by examining the inside of the throat.

- **Lymphoma and leukemia** The lymphocytes of the immune system itself can occasionally become cancerous, causing either lymphoma or leukemia. Swollen lymph nodes can occur anywhere in the body and gradually enlarge over several months. In this case, there are no signs of primary infection or cancer, and a lymph node biopsy may be the only way of making the diagnosis.

THROMBOSIS
The blocking of a blood vessel by a blood clot, or thrombus.

What are the causes?
Abnormal blood clotting is sometimes a consequence of diseases of the blood vessels, generally the arteries. The arteries are usually damaged by atheroma (arteriosclerosis), caused by smoking, diabetes, high blood pressure, or high cholesterol levels. When arteries are blocked by thrombosis, the local tissues are unable to get enough oxygen and will eventually die. This can cause clots in the brain (stroke), the heart (coronary thrombosis, myocardial infarction), or the legs (gangrene).

Blood clots in veins are often caused by an increase in the tendency of the blood to clot, for example in women taking the contraceptive pill or during pregnancy. Blood also has a tendency to clot if you are immobile for too long. This is the cause of the so-called "economy class syndrome" and of clots after operations.

Blood clots in veins generally start in the legs, where they cause pain and swelling in the calves; this is referred to as deep venous thrombosis (DVT). Sometimes these clots break off and travel through the veins to the lungs. Big clots can then damage the blood supply to the lungs, leading to breathlessness, coughing up blood, and pains in the chest.

How is it diagnosed?
A doctor may diagnose superficial clots from a description of the discomfort and an examination of the skin. DVT can be diagnosed either by ultrasound or through injecting a contrast dye into a large vein in the foot or ankle. An X-ray may then detect clots.

What are the treatment options?
During prolonged periods of immobility, such as after surgery or when someone is on a long flight, clotting can be prevented by exercising the legs regularly. If correctly used, elastic stockings can help to make clotting less likely.

A superficial clot may respond positively to heat, elevation, and aspirin or NSAIDs. DVT is normally treated by injection of an anticoagulant, such as heparin, to prevent clots from growing. After heparin treatment, warfarin may be prescribed for several months to thin the blood. Sometimes, a drug is needed to aid the body in dissolving the clot. Support tights may be recommended to prevent swelling and reduce the chances of complications.

TIREDNESS
This is the normal response of the body to an excess of activity—physical or mental—and not enough sleep.

It can be very difficult to distinguish normal tiredness from excessive tiredness. People who are tired even after eight hours of sleep every night may have an underlying problem.

What are the causes?
Fatigue is common in people who have infections, and it may take several weeks to get over the excessive tiredness caused by a bad case of the flu. Many diseases can cause excessive tiredness, and it is often seen in people who have anemia, arthritis, and cancer. If these diseases are ruled out, the tiredness may be caused by chronic fatigue syndrome (p. 140), also known as myalgic encephalitis.

One in five men and one in three women admit feeling tired "most of the time."

How is it diagnosed?
Patients with chronic fatigue syndrome may also have pain in the muscles, sore throats, and other symptoms.

What are the treatment options?
Once the underlying cause has been established, the appropriate treatment can be determined.

WEIGHT LOSS
The loss of more than five to seven pounds can suggest that there may be underlying disease.

What are the causes?
Psychological issues or problems with either the upper or lower parts of the gastrointestinal tract can all cause weight loss. If none of these is present, weight loss may be the result of a wide range of other disorders including hormone problems, infections, and tumors.

Loss of appetite is common in upper gastrointestinal tract diseases and psychological disorders. If the patient has persistent diarrhea, it may suggest problems with the lower intestinal tract.

What are the treatment options?
Treatment will depend on the underlying cause of the weight loss.

DISEASES AND DISORDERS

ANTIBODY DEFICIENCY
A lack of adequate antibodies to protect the body from disease.

Antibodies are proteins produced in the blood to counteract the effect of toxins produced by bacteria.

What are the causes?
Antibody deficiency can be caused by an underlying disease, for example chronic lymphocytic leukemia or myeloma, particularly in older people. It can also be genetic in origin, in which case it can affect young people. Whatever the cause, the consequences are the same.

What are the symptoms?
Antibodies are most important in protecting the airways, from the nose to the lungs. These parts of the body are particularly exposed to bacteria and viruses in the air. People with antibody deficiency tend to suffer repeated infections of the airways, resulting in runny noses, sinusitis (the sinuses are air spaces in the skull on either side of the nose), sore throats, and chest infections. After one infection has gone away, another soon follows. Cases of pneumonia are common, and some patients have infections of the bones or joints, or meningitis.

How is it diagnosed?
Antibody deficiency is easy to diagnose by checking the patient's immunoglobulin levels (p. 110). Unfortunately, there is often a delay of several years before the correct diagnosis is made.

What are the treatment options?
Immunologists usually treat patients with antibody deficiency, because treatment can be very complicated and is likely to be required for the remainder of the patient's life. Some people with mild forms of the illness respond well to lifelong antibiotics. Other sufferers need to have immunoglobulin replacement therapy. Immunoglobulin can be extracted from donor blood and needs to be given by injection; it can be given intravenously, usually every three weeks, or into the skin (subcutaneously) once a week. This treatment continues for the rest of the patient's life. To make the treatment more convenient, patients may be trained to give themselves immunoglobulin at home.

Antibody deficiency can be one type of primary immune deficiency, along with severe combined immunodeficiency (SCID, see p. 151), complement deficiency, and chronic granulomatous disease. In the U.S., there are many local, national, and online support organizations, including the Immune Deficiency Foundation at www.primaryimmune.org.

AUTOIMMUNE DISEASES
In autoimmunity, the immune system attacks the body's own cells and tissues.

There are many different autoimmune disorders, including some of the most common diseases. Some important ones are shown below; many of these are mentioned in sections of this book or in other books in the series.

The purpose of T cells and B cells in the immune system is to attack bacteria, viruses, and other alien microbes that enter the body. The immune system has mechanisms for preventing it from attacking normal components of the

Autoimmune diseases

DISEASE	WHAT IS ATTACKED BY THE IMMUNE SYSTEM
Type I diabetes	Insulin-secreting cells in the pancreas
Thyroid disease (Graves' disease, Hashimoto's disease)	Thyroid gland
Immune thrombocytopenia (ITP)	Platelets in the blood
Rheumatoid arthritis	Joint linings and other tissues
Systemic lupus erythematosus (SLE)	Joints, skin, kidneys
Pernicious anemia	Cells lining the stomach
Celiac disease	The lining of the small intestine
Multiple sclerosis	White matter in the brain and spinal cord

body. As T cells and B cells develop, they are "educated"—in the thymus and bone marrow, respectively—not to attack normal body tissues. Autoimmune diseases develop when this training process goes wrong.

What are the causes?
The training process can go wrong for genetic reasons, so autoimmunity often tends to run through families. It is not unusual, for example, for one sibling to have thyroid disease and another to have diabetes. Sometimes the abnormal genes can cause an unlucky person to have more than one autoimmune disease. Other factors, such as infections and sometimes drugs, can trigger autoimmunity in people who have the relevant genes.

How is it diagnosed?
Autoimmune diseases are diagnosed by investigations that show that organs being attacked are not working. For example, in pernicious anemia, it is possible to show that the intestine is not absorbing enough vitamin B_{12}. It is then also possible to show that the immune system is making antibodies against the stomach lining cells that enable the absorption of vitamin B_{12}. These autoantibody tests are available for many autoimmune diseases.

What are the treatment options?
For some diseases, it is simplest to replace the products of the tissues that have been damaged by the immune system. For instance, diabetic patients may be given insulin, and people with autoimmune thyroid disease may be given the thyroid hormone thyroxine. In other cases, it is necessary to prevent the immune system from causing further damage. This can be done using immunosuppressive drugs, which try to "turn off" the immune system. These include steroids (prednisolone), azathioprine, infliximab, methotrexate, and cyclosporin. Each of these drugs has a range of side effects, but they all turn off the normal immune response to bacteria and viruses. Patients who are on these drugs are therefore at higher risk of infection.

BLEEDING DISORDERS
These disorders occur when the mechanisms for making the blood clot are not working.

What are the causes?
Platelets are small cells in the blood that stick together whenever a blood vessel is damaged—such as when the skin is cut. If there are insufficient platelets in the blood, the blood will not clot. This can happen if the bone marrow has been damaged so that not enough platelets are being produced, for example in leukemia. It can also happen when platelets are destroyed by diseases such as immune thrombocytopenia, ITP (p. 146).

Proteins in the blood also help the blood clot during injuries. These proteins, called clotting factors, are produced mainly in the liver, so if a patient has severe liver disease, the blood will not clot.

Some males are unable to produce one clotting factor, factor VIII, because they have inherited an abnormal gene for the protein; this is known as hemophilia (p. 144). Without treatment, these males bleed too heavily.

Alternatively, the clotting factors can be triggered abnormally by infections. Clotting then takes place in healthy, uninjured blood vessels. All the clotting factors are then used up, and there is bleeding elsewhere.

How is it diagnosed?
Platelet deficiency can be diagnosed by doing a complete blood count, and all these problems can be diagnosed by means of a clotting screen.

What are the treatment options?
Drugs can be administered to control excessive bleeding in some patients; others need transfusions of plasma products. Lifelong treatment is normally required.

BONE MARROW FAILURE
The bone marrow is a factory for producing blood cells. Its failure is defined as an inability to produce adequate numbers of blood cells.

Bone marrow produces neutrophils (for fighting infection), red cells (for carrying oxygen around the body), and platelets (which help the blood to clot). Every day the bone marrow stem cells divide to produce many billions of each cell type. If the bone marrow is damaged, it cannot produce the necessary blood cells.

What are the causes?
Damage can be caused by diseases of the bone marrow cells, such as leukemia, lymphoma, or other cancers; in these cases, the normal marrow is simply squeezed out by the malignant cells. In other cases, the marrow fails because it is damaged by drugs, radiation, or the immune system.

This can be referred to as aplastic anemia, which occurs as a result of an autoimmune attack on the marrow.

Drug damage is the commonest cause of bone marrow failure. It can happen as a result of cytotoxic chemotherapy drugs used to treat cancers, when the risk of bone marrow failure is related to the dose of chemotherapy given. This is because these drugs aim to prevent cells from dividing, making damage to bone marrow is almost inevitable.

Very rarely, other drugs, for example some antibiotics, can cause bone marrow failure. Such reactions are very unlikely and are totally unpredictable. Finally, exposure to certain chemicals, including benzene, insecticides, and heavy metals, may cause bone marrow failure.

What are the symptoms?
Anemia, frequent infections, and unexplained bleeding are all symptoms of bone marrow failure.

How is it diagnosed?
Bone marrow failure may be suggested by a complete blood count test. To be absolutely certain that this is what is wrong when a patient shows very low blood counts, the bone marrow must be examined. This is done by bone marrow aspiration, which involves removing a little marrow fluid via a needle, for microscopic evaluation.

A bone marrow biopsy (see p. 108) may be performed at the same time as bone marrow aspiration. Bone marrow aspiration involves sucking out bone marrow, whereas a bone marrow biopsy involves taking out a core of bone marrow and solid bone. The biopsy provides additional useful information regarding possible abnormalities in the bone marrow that are not always revealed by aspiration. A biopsy may show cancer cells if they exist. In the aplastic anemia types of problem (caused by drugs, chemical, or autoimmune disease), it is possible to see that there is a massive reduction of the blood-manufacturing cells.

What are the treatment options?
Because of all the complications, bone marrow failure is a serious problem. Patients are usually admitted to the hospital so that they can be closely monitored. Patients with a very low neutrophil count, for example, need to have their temperature taken frequently, because a raised temperature is one of the earliest signs of infection.

If there is evidence of cancer, this must be treated. Exposure to drugs and chemicals that cause bone marrow failure must be checked. If there is evidence of an autoimmune attack on the marrow, immunosuppressive drugs may be given.

Much of the treatment for bone marrow failure is supportive. For example, blood transfusions can be given to relieve the symptoms of patients with severe anemia, and platelets can be given to people who are bleeding because of low platelet counts. The hope is that whatever caused the bone marrow to fail in the first place will improve. When improvement is very unlikely, a stem cell transplant may be carried out if there is a suitable donor available (p. 120).

BURKITT'S LYMPHOMA
A particular kind of lymphoma of the B cells, Burkitt's lymphoma also belongs to the group of non-Hodgkin's lymphomas.

This disease has a higher incidence in equatorial Africa than in the rest of the world, and it was in Africa that surgeon Dennis Burkitt first noticed that the tumor often occurred in the jaw. In the rest of the world, it is usually first found in the abdomen.

What are the causes?
This lymphoma is commonly associated with the presence of the Epstein-Barr virus, a kind of herpes virus that causes infectious mononucleosis (p. 147) and that most people harbor; the tumor is more common in children than in adults. Why it occasionally causes cancer is not known.

What are the symptoms?
A tumor on the jaw causes pain and swelling and loosening of the teeth; an abdominal tumor causes local pain and swelling. The spread to other sites may be rapid.

How is it diagnosed?
Diagnosis will be confirmed by biopsy of the lump and examination of the biopsy tissue under the microscope. This will reveal the characteristic diffuse malignant B cells, which do not look like normal B cells.

What are the treatment options?
Burkitt's lymphoma responds well to chemotherapy, and prolonged remissions can be achieved with this kind of treatment. Facial tumors tend to respond better than abdominal tumors. Surgery is also an option.

CHRONIC FATIGUE SYNDROME
Extreme tiredness, which does not improve with sleep and is made worse by physical or mental exertion.

This condition is also called myalgic encephalitis (ME).

What is the cause?
The cause of chronic fatigue syndrome (CFS) is not known. Because the illness has been found to affect people in clusters, for example groups of people working at the same place, some researchers have thought that it is triggered by a specific infection. However, no triggering infection has been found consistently in everyone suffering from CFS. The idea that infection may cause CFS has led some doctors to think that the immune system is involved in causing the symptoms of CFS. To date there is no evidence of immunological problems in all patients with CFS.

HELP YOUR DOCTOR HELP YOU

Choosing a CFS support group
Because chronic fatigue syndrome is so poorly understood, it is important to find a doctor who is sympathetic and informed if you are diagnosed with the condition. Many sufferers also find joining a support group useful. Most support groups are free or charge only a small membership fee. A good support group should

- *Be well established, with a track record of meeting its members' needs.*

- *Include people with whom you feel comfortable, who will neither dominate discussions nor keep silent.*

- *Have a good mix of the newly diagnosed and those with longer-standing illness, so that there is a wealth of different experiences and perceptions on which to draw.*

Groups to avoid, on the other hand, include those that

- *Advocate that you stop taking prescribed medication.*

- *Offer a quick fix to the problem.*

- *Try to persuade sufferers to purchase "miracle" cures.*

What are the symptoms?
The most obvious symptom of chronic fatigue syndrome is extreme tiredness, but many patients have other symptoms, such as muscle pain or sore throats, that may develop after an infection and tend to last many months or even years. Although many people with CFS become depressed, the current thinking is that this is a result, not the cause, of all the other symptoms. In other words, CFS is not primarily a psychological illness.

How is it diagnosed?
There is no specific test for CFS. The diagnosis is made in patients who have all the symptoms with no other explanation for them. For example, it is important to rule out anemia as a cause of chronic fatigue.

Many patients with CFS feel that the medical profession does not take their symptoms seriously, and one of the best things that can happen to CFS patients is to find a medical team that believes their symptoms are real and wants to try to improve them. Patients also find it helpful to be told that in most cases, their symptoms will improve over time.

What are the treatment options?
Because it is not understood what causes CFS, there is currently no cure. Treatment aims to improve the fatigue, usually by encouraging people to gradually build up their tolerance of exercise. Patients may be given a series of graded exercises that they build up over several weeks or months. For example, they may be asked to walk 150 feet a day in the first week, 300 feet a day the second week, and so on.

Because depression is such a common part of CFS, many patients also benefit from input from psychologists or, sometimes, antidepressant drugs.

CHRONIC GRANULOMATOUS DISEASE
A rare type of inherited immune deficiency affecting the neutrophils—blood cells that fight infection.

What is the cause?
Patients suffering from chronic granulomatous disease (CGD) are able to make neutrophils—the most prevalent white blood cell type—but the neutrophils are usually unable to kill bacteria. Normally, a few neutrophils are recruited to the site of an infection by immune system signals and they then kill the bacteria. Once the neutrophils have done their work, they die.

What are the symptoms?

Once the immune system is responding to infection, pus (an accumulation of dead neutrophils) is usually produced in small amounts at the site of the infection. In CGD, because the neutrophils are unable to kill the bacteria, they continue to accumulate and a large amount of pus forms, resulting in an abscess.

How is it diagnosed?

Confirmation of the diagnosis is done by specialty laboratory analysis, which looks at the function of the blood cells and the cells' metabolism.

What are the treatment options?

Patients with CGD are given antibiotics to clear or prevent infections. Stem cell transplant and gene therapy are currently being tested as treatments for CGD.

COMPLEMENT DEFICIENCIES

A rare type of inherited immune deficiency.

Complement is blood protein, which plays a role in the immune system's fight against infection. Some people inherit mutations in their complement genes, making them very prone to infections, particularly types of meningitis. Some people with complement deficiencies are also more likely to develop the autoimmune disease systemic lupus erythematosus, SLE (p. 154).

What are the symptoms?

Symptoms depend on the specific complement deficiency. Some people remain symptomless. Those who suffer from frequent infections may develop fever, headaches, diarrhea, and chest pain. If an autoimmune condition develops, a patient may lose weight and suffer from a rash and joint pain. Other symptoms include pain, swelling of the face, and lumps on the skin.

How is it diagnosed?

Blood tests measure the activity of the complement system and identify those parts that are not working properly. Specific tests for the individual components of the system are then carried out, as well as a white blood cell count.

What are the treatment options?

At present, there is no way to cure complement deficiency. Any resulting infections can be treated with antibiotics, and patients can be vaccinated to reduce the risks of diseases such as the flu and pneumonia. A bone marrow transplant is appropriate in some cases.

Some patients remain healthy; others suffer frequent infections requiring hospital stays. Those with autoimmune diseases can have a normal life expectancy, but some types of complement deficiency have a high death rate, with few patients still alive ten years after diagnosis.

DIABETES MELLITUS

A condition in which glucose is not broken down to produce energy because of a lack of the pancreatic hormone insulin or an inability of the tissues to respond to insulin's effects.

This relatively common condition results in persistently high levels of glucose in the blood, because the cells are unable to absorb glucose from the bloodstream as they normally would. When the sugar level becomes very high, there can be damage to the blood vessels (atheroma, arteriosclerosis), increasing the risk of problems such as stroke, gangrene, and coronary thrombosis. The high blood sugar level also damages the eyes and kidneys.

There are two types of diabetes, type I and type II. The cause of a case of diabetes is usually not known.

Type I diabetes

This is an autoimmune disease. Like other autoimmune diseases, it tends to run in families and usually starts in children, who rapidly become ill. They lose weight dramatically, and if they are not treated with insulin, will go into a coma. When a patient first becomes ill, there are signs that the body is producing antibodies that act against the islet cells in the pancreas that normally secrete insulin. These antibodies can be tested for in the laboratory. The immune attack on the pancreas doesn't take long to destroy the islet cells; once this happens, the antibodies disappear.

Type II diabetes

This type of diabetes affects older people. Various factors in addition to increasing age put people at risk; obesity is thought to be a major factor in the development of the disease, and affected individuals are usually overweight. This form of the disease is not thought to be autoimmune, but it also tends to run in families. People with type II diabetes are still able to produce some insulin, unlike those with type I diabetes.

What are the symptoms?

Type I diabetes usually appears suddenly, with children complaining of excessive thirst and dry mouth; there is excessive urination, dramatic weight loss, and possibly coma.

Type II diabetes is often only picked up when sugar is detected in the urine or raised sugar levels are detected in the blood. Patients may complain of a lack of energy and simply feeling "off."

How is it diagnosed?

Diagnosis is usually made on the basis of raised glucose levels in the blood.

What are the treatment options?

People with type I diabetes need insulin treatment for the rest of their lives. This involves injections, which patients are taught to give themselves, often several times a day. Immunologists are looking at other ways of preventing or treating this type of diabetes. If a patient is diagnosed before the islet cells are destroyed, immunosuppressive drugs may prevent the disease; this has been tested in clinical trials. While children are on immunosuppressive drugs, diabetes can be prevented, but, as soon as the drugs are stopped (which they eventually have to be because of potential side effects) the immune system starts attacking the pancreas, and diabetes develops. Another immunological treatment is a pancreas transplant. This is being tested in trials on patients who already have diabetes.

Many patients with type II diabetes do not need insulin injections. Instead, the condition is controlled by sticking to a low-sugar diet, losing any excess weight, or taking tablets to lower the blood sugar levels. The outlook for these patients is good.

GRAVES' DISEASE

Autoimmune disease that causes overactivity of the thyroid gland—hyperthyroidism.

What are the causes?

In Graves' disease, the immune system makes antibodies against the thyroid gland, stimulating it to secrete increased amounts of thyroxine. The thyroid gland is not damaged by this process, but it does become larger than normal.

What are the symptoms?

The thyroid overactivity causes weight loss and restlessness. A special characteristic of patients with Graves' disease is that they have very prominent eyes. This happens because of a buildup of tissue behind the eyes, not because the eyes are swollen.

Graves' disease affects only 0.25 percent of the population overall, but it is eight times more common in women than men.

How is it diagnosed?

Graves' disease is diagnosed by performing thyroid function tests and tests of autoimmunity.

What are the treatment options?

Treatment consists of anti-thyroid medication to reduce the activity of the thyroid gland.

HASHIMOTO'S DISEASE

In contrast to Graves' disease, this autoimmune disease causes underactivity of the thyroid—hypothyroidism.

Hashimoto's disease is a typical autoimmune disease. In this case, the immune system attacks the thyroid gland, resulting in its gradual destruction.

What are the symptoms?

The thyroid gland may initially be swollen. Underactivity of the thyroid causes weight gain and decreased energy.

How is it diagnosed?

Hashimoto's disease is diagnosed through thyroid function tests and autoimmunity tests.

What are the treatment options?

Treatment consists of thyroxine tablets to replace the hormones that the thyroid should be making. Medication and regular blood tests should keep symptoms under control and mean that there are no long-term effects.

HEMOLYTIC ANEMIAS

Anemias resulting from hemolysis—the excessive destruction of red blood cells.

Red blood cells have a limited life span of about 120 days. When they are showing signs of damage, they are taken up by cells in the spleen and destroyed. The body recycles some of the valuable components of the red cells, such as iron, whereas others, for example the yellow pigment bilirubin, are disposed of in the liver.

A number of different mechanisms can damage red cells, and the damage may be great enough to destroy those in the circulation or to cause them to be taken up by the spleen.

What are the causes?
Hemolysis can be caused by certain genetic diseases; by some infections, such as malaria; or by the immune system attacking the red blood cells.

- **Hereditary spherocytosis** In this genetic disease, the red cells have an abnormal shape and form spheres instead of discs. The spleen takes up all the sphere-shaped red cells, so sufferers have bouts of anemia.
- **Sickle cell disease** This is another inherited problem that can cause anemia (p. 134).
- **Malaria** In this case, the parasite lives inside the red cells. As it grows, it damages the red cells, which are eventually destroyed in the circulation of blood in the spleen.
- **Blood of the wrong type** If the wrong type of blood is given during a transfusion, antibodies will bind on to the red cells and activate the complement, a constituent of the blood (p. 141). One of the roles of complement is to punch holes in invading bacteria, but if complement is activated in the vicinity of red cells, it punches holes in those. The cells rapidly burst, and there are two major consequences: First, there are fewer cells to transport oxygen around the body, resulting in anemia; second, the cells' contents are also released into the circulation, where they can cause damage including kidney failure.
- **Hemolytic disease of the newborn** This is similar in some ways to a transfusion of the wrong blood. The red cells are the unborn baby's own cells and the antibody, which in this instance comes from the mother, is nearly always against the Rhesus system.
- **Auto immune hemolytic anemia** It is possible for the immune system to attack the body's own normal red blood cells in a form of autoimmunity. Effects can be dramatic if the cells are destroyed rapidly in the circulation. More frequently, there is a gradual attack on the red cells, which are prematurely taken up by the spleen. Autoimmune hemolytic anemia can occur as a result of other diseases—for example, it is sometimes seen in cases of chronic lymphatic leukemia (p. 148), or systemic lupus erythematosus, SLE (p. 154). Sometimes drugs, such as penicillin, can trigger autoimmune hemolytic anemia.

What are the symptoms?
Symptoms of hemolysis are the same as those of anemia: fatigue, breathlessness, and palpitations. The patient may be very pale or slightly jaundiced. In this case, the jaundice is caused by excessive amounts of bilirubin in the bloodstream and not liver disease. Some patients, particularly those with autoimmune hemolytic anemia, have an enlarged spleen.

How is it diagnosed?
A diagnosis of hemolytic anemia is suggested by finding reduced hemoglobin levels in the blood count. Sometimes the blood film (p. 105) is very useful. For example, in hereditary spherocytosis, the abnormal sphere-shaped red cells are apparent. In cases where the immune system is attacking red cells, Coombs' test (p. 106) will show that antibodies are binding on to cells.

What are the treatment options?
The treatment of hemolytic anemia depends on the cause. When there is severe hemolysis, it is important to keep the patient well hydrated so that the toxic substances released during destruction of the red cells pass out through the kidneys. If the anemia is severe, it may be necessary to give a blood transfusion; this is done with great care.

In the hereditary disorders (but not sickle cell disease), it may be necessary to remove the spleen through surgery (a splenectomy) to control the anemia. The decision to do this always has to be balanced against the risk that the body will lose some of its ability to fight infection.

In cases of autoimmune hemolytic anemia, immunosuppressive drugs may be given. If these do not work, it is sometimes necessary to remove the spleen.

HEMOLYTIC DISEASE OF THE NEWBORN
In this disease, a pregnant woman's immune system attacks the baby's red blood cells, causing severe anemia.

For this to happen, the mother and baby must have different Rhesus blood groups: The mother must be Rhesus negative and the baby Rhesus positive because it has inherited the positive gene from its father.

What are the causes?
The Rhesus positive gene makes the baby's red cells different from the mother's. If a few of the baby's red cells

leak into the mother's circulation during pregnancy or labor, her immune system will recognize them as being different and will start making antibodies. These antibodies usually do not cause problems for the first Rhesus positive baby, but if the mother becomes pregnant with another Rhesus positive baby, the amount of antibodies increases. These will cross the placenta into the baby's circulation, and the unborn child's red cells are attacked as a result.

What are the symptoms?
The baby is born severely anemic, and a positive result in a Coombs' test (p. 106) will indicate that the baby's red cells have been attacked by antibodies.

What are the treatment options?
A severely anemic baby may require an exchange blood transfusion, in which its blood is exchanged with fresh blood. Anemia in the newborn can, however, be prevented. Only a minority of women are Rhesus negative, and they can be identified by blood type testing during pregnancy. After each baby is born, the mother can be given an injection of Anti D, which works by rapidly destroying any red cells from the baby that have leaked into the mother's circulation. Once these are destroyed, the mother's immune system will no longer be stimulated to make anti-Rhesus antibodies.

HEMOPHILIA
An X-linked inherited disorder of the clotting system that only affects males.

What are the causes?
Hemophiliacs have a mutation in the gene for factor VIII, one of the proteins that normally helps the blood to clot. (See also X-linked disorders, p. 155.)

What are the symptoms?
Because of this disorder of the clotting system, hemophiliacs tend to bleed heavily after even minor injuries. Most of this bleeding takes place internally, often into joints. Over the years, this damages the joints, and hemophiliacs can end up very disabled.

How is it diagnosed?
Hemophilia is easily diagnosed by doing a clotting screen and then measuring the levels of factor VIII.

What are the treatment options?
Hemophilia is treatable with factor VIII. Patients are usually trained so that they can give themselves factor VIII intravenously at home.

Factor VIII can be extracted from donated blood, but in order to manufacture sufficient factor VIII, blood from many different donors must be pooled. This carries a risk of spreading infections by bloodborne viruses, particularly HIV and hepatitis C, which attacks the liver. In the early 1980s, many hemophiliacs across the world were infected with these viruses, but since the mid-1980s, blood has been tested for HIV, and tests for hepatitis C were introduced in the 1990s. Factor VIII manufactured from donated blood should now be much safer.

Factor VIII can also be manufactured using DNA technology. The human gene for factor VIII is inserted into bacterial cells, which then produce factor VIII protein; this technology produces factor VIII that is free from the risk of infection. Known as recombinant factor VIII, this type is very expensive, but hemophilia organizations around the world are trying to make sure that patients receive it.

HIV INFECTION/AIDS
HIV is the virus that can cause AIDS—acquired immunodeficiency syndrome.

The HIV (human immunodeficiency virus) epidemic started in the 1980s, when it received considerable publicity. AIDS may have dropped out of the headlines in the West, but it has not disappeared: Over the past ten years, it has killed tens of millions of people and orphaned millions of children.

What are the causes?
The HIV virus infects and damages the T helper cells—known as the CD4 cells—in the immune system. These cells, which coordinate the immune response to bacteria, viruses, parasites, and cancer, have been described as the conductors of the immunological orchestra. When T helper cells are not working, the immune system is unable to respond to infections and cancers.

HIV spreads from person to person with intimate contact. This includes penetrative vaginal or anal sex between men and women or men and men. Oral sex can also transmit the virus, but this is not as prevalent. HIV can also be spread by drug users who share needles and can pass from mother to baby in the womb, during childbirth, or by breastfeeding. HIV is now rarely spread by blood transfusions.

What are the symptoms?

The majority of people do not even know when they have been infected with HIV, but in about 10 percent of patients, there can be a shortlived illness, with sore throat, fever, and rashes. HIV takes a long time to damage the T helper cells. It typically takes about five years before the infected patient notices any symptoms at all.

Early symptoms of immune system damage caused by HIV infection include fungal infections of the mouth and severe attacks of herpes or chicken pox. Other patients notice weight loss and lymphadenopathy—swollen lymph nodes (p. 135).

Specific infections and cancers are characteristic of AIDS. As the immune deficiency worsens, more severe infections occur. These include specific types of chest infection, for example pneumocystis pneumonia and tuberculosis. Later on, vision may be damaged by a virus called CMV, and the parasite *Toxoplasma gondii* may cause toxoplasmosis, which can lead to brain abscesses. The severe immune system weakness may allow cancers to grow unchecked. These include non-Hodgkin's lymphoma and a skin cancer known as Kaposi's sarcoma. As time goes by, it is typical for patients to have several different infections and possibly one of the forms of cancer.

Nearly one third of all adults in the U.S. and Europe have antibodies to Toxoplasma, which means they have been exposed to this parasite.

How is it diagnosed?

Blood tests can show if HIV is active and damaging the immune system. The viral load test is a type of polymerase chain reaction (PCR) test (p. 109), which measures how actively HIV is dividing, and CD4 counts show how much damage HIV has done to these cells. Over the years, the viral load tends to increase, and the CD4 count falls.

What are the treatment options?

Each of the individual infections and cancers can usually be treated. Once an infection has been cured, patients remain on antibiotics to prevent the infection from coming back, as it will very likely do when the immune system is weakened. When a patient has several different infections at the same time, treatment becomes much more difficult.

The best way to treat HIV infection is to prevent the damage from occurring in the first place. Antiretroviral drugs (p. 112) prevent HIV from going through its life cycle and damaging T helper cells. These drugs can be taken once the viral load is showing signs of high HIV activity and the CD4 count is beginning to fall.

One problem with HIV is that the virus mutates continuously. It is possible for it to become resistant to the antiretroviral drugs. Patients usually take a combination of three or even four different antiretroviral drugs because the chances of the virus becoming resistant to three or four different drugs at once is less likely than to one drug alone.

Millions of dollars have been spent on vaccine research for HIV, so far without much success. One reason is that there is no suitable animal on which vaccines can be tested. In the past, vaccines have been tested initially on animals and then tried out on humans. Chimpanzees are the only animals other than humans that are attacked by HIV, but scientists and others are reluctant to use chimpanzees in vaccine experiments because they are a protected species.

Another problem is that there are hundreds of strains of HIV. Because the virus mutates so quickly, it is highly likely that an HIV strain from Africa would be very different from a strain from North America. A vaccine that works for an African strain would probably not work for a European strain and vice versa.

What is the outlook?

People infected with HIV may remain well for ten years or more, but at present it is considered likely that the vast majority, if not all, will eventually develop AIDS. Long-term use of recently introduced drugs may improve this outlook. Improvements in treatment of infections, as well new drugs, mean that many people remain physically and mentally healthy for years after HIV has been diagnosed.

HODGKIN'S DISEASE
A tumor of the lymphatic tissue that is classified separately from non-Hodgkin's lymphomas (NHL).

Hodgkin's disease (HD) is more common in males than females. It occurs mainly in young adults, with a second peak in middle age.

What are the causes?

The cause is unknown. An association with the Epstein-Barr virus (which causes infectious mononucleosis) has been suggested but not unequivocally proven.

What are the symptoms?

A patient with HD may have painless swollen lymph nodes, possibly associated with general tiredness, fever, itchiness, night sweats, and weight loss. Generalized itching or pain in enlarged lymph nodes after drinking alcohol is also an occasional symptom. A common site for an HD tumor is in the chest between the lungs; this may cause a cough or painful breathing.

How is it diagnosed?
Investigations to confirm HD include
- a blood test, which may show anemia. The test will also check for other diseases that may cause swollen lymph nodes, such as infectious mononucleosis;
- a bone marrow biopsy, done to exclude other hematological disorders, but HD is rare in bone marrow; and
- a chest X-ray, which will show any swollen nodes in this region. Swollen nodes will be biopsied and examined for the presence of cells characteristic of HD.

What are the treatment options?
Depending on the stage the disease has reached, treatment will be either radiation alone or radiation with chemotherapy. The management of Hodgkin's disease is one of the success stories in cancer research, and most cases can now be cured. However, this success has been tempered by the discovery that the high-dose therapies needed to cure this disease may actually cause secondary malignancy, such as leukemia, later in life. One aim of cancer therapy research is to tailor the treatment dose according to the volume of disease, cell, and cytogenetic subtype. It may then be possible to reduce the chances of the therapy causing another cancer, while also avoiding an underdose with potential for relapse.

IMMUNE DEFICIENCIES
Although there are many types of immune deficiencies, they all result in vulnerability to infection.

Immune deficiencies can be caused by relatively rare genetic problems, such as severe combined immunodeficiency (SCID, p. 151), chronic granulomatous disease (CGD, p. 140), and complement and antibody deficiency. Immune deficiencies can also be caused by drugs; for example, most cases of neutropenia (a decrease in the number of neutrophils in the blood) are caused by cytotoxic drugs used for cancer treatment. Immunosuppressive drugs used to treat autoimmune disease or to support organ transplantation also cause immune deficiency, but the biggest cause worldwide is HIV infection (p. 144).

More than 80 immunodeficiency diseases are currently recognized by the World Health Organization.

What are the treatment options?
Some types of immunodeficiency respond to treatment with intravenous gammaglobulin (IVIG); in others, stem cell transplant may be an option. Antibiotics are prescribed to treat the recurrent infections.

IMMUNE THROMBOCYTOPENIA
An autoimmune bleeding disorder, immune thrombocytopenia leads to destruction of the platelets in the blood.

Platelets are the blood cells that play a part in the blood clotting process following injury. If the platelets are being destroyed, there is a tendency for bleeding to take place. Patients with immune thrombocytopenia (ITP) make antibodies against their own platelets. The spleen is responsible for clearing old red cells, white cells, and platelets from the blood. In ITP, the platelets coated with antibodies are destroyed by the spleen.

What are the causes?
There are two main types of ITP. In children, the disease tends to be triggered by infection. Childhood ITP may be quite severe, but after a few weeks the platelet count generally returns to normal.

Adult ITP tends to be a long-lasting disease that may continue for the rest of the patient's life. Sometimes patients have an underlying problem, such as SLE (p. 154) or chronic lymphocytic leukemia (p. 148).

What are the symptoms?
Patients with ITP first notice abnormal bruising or bleeding. The doctor may notice that the spleen is enlarged.

How is it diagnosed?
The low numbers of platelets in the blood can be diagnosed by a complete blood count. Sometimes a bone marrow examination needs to be done to confirm that the problem is caused by destruction of platelets rather than impaired production of platelets, which is part of bone marrow failure (p. 138).

What are the treatment options?
There are many different treatments for ITP. If the platelet count is very low or if the patient has serious bleeding, it is possible to give platelet transfusions from donated blood. More common, treatment aims to stop platelet destruction

by using immunosuppressive drugs (see autoimmune diseases, p. 137), intravenous immunoglobulin (see antibody deficiency, p. 137), or Anti D injections (see hemolytic disease of the newborn, p. 143). In some cases, ITP cannot be controlled by these measures, and the removal of the spleen is the only way to stop it destroying platelet cells.

IMMUNOGLOBULIN A (IGA) DEFICIENCY
This is the most common antibody deficiency.

IgA is the antibody found in all body secretions: for example in saliva, in feces, and in tears and mucus in the chest. IgA in breast milk is an important source of antibodies for babies. IgA deficiency is not life-threatening, but people who do not produce IgA may have a higher risk of infections of the chest and intestine.

INFECTIOUS MONONUCLEOSIS
This is a viral infection.

What are the causes?
The Epstein-Barr virus, one of the herpes viruses, is the cause of infectious mononucleosis. It commonly affects children and young people between ages 15 and 25. It is not particularly infectious and is contracted by intimate contact, such as kissing, with someone infected with the virus, which is carried by a large percentage of the population. The incubation period can be as long as six weeks after infection.

What are the symptoms?
The disease usually starts with a sore throat and fever, tiredness, and a feeling of being unwell. The lymph nodes in the neck, armpits, and groin become swollen. Sometimes there is a rash. In severe cases, the spleen may be enlarged. On the other hand, many people who become infected with the Epstein-Barr virus experience no symptoms at all.

How is it diagnosed?
The doctor takes account of all the symptoms, and a blood test confirms the diagnosis by showing the presence in the blood of antibodies to the Epstein-Barr virus and also of characteristic B cells.

What are the treatment options?
The patient can take painkillers to relieve fever and pain, but rest is generally all the treatment that is needed. Most people recover fully within four to six weeks, although a feeling of fatigue can persist for several more weeks.

LEUKEMIA
Cancer of the white blood cells, which can affect any of the white blood cell types.

Lymphoblastic leukemia is cancer of B or T lymphocytes or their precursor cells (immature B or T cells). Myeloid leukemia is cancer of another type of cell produced in the bone marrow, for example, neutrophils.

Children are mainly affected by acute lymphoblastic leukemia (ALL) or acute myeloid leukemia (AML), which are usually aggressive, fast-growing tumors if untreated, and by chronic myeloid (or myelogenous) leukemia (CML), which begins as a slowly progressing disease but usually terminates with an acute phase. The most common leukemias found in adults are AML and chronic lymphocytic leukemia (CLL), a type which has a much slower course. All leukemias affect the bone marrow (where cells are usually first seen). CLL can affect the lymph nodes and is thus similar to lymphoma.

What are the causes?
The cause of leukemia is known only in a small number of instances. Some cases of T cell leukemia are induced by a virus, Human T cell Leukemia Virus-1 (HTLV-1), which is rare outside Japan and the Caribbean. Acute myeloid leukemia may be caused by high doses of chemotherapy and radiation that have been given as treatment for previous cancers such as Hodgkin's disease.

What are the symptoms?
In children, the first signs may be loss of energy, tiredness, and fever. There may be persistent infections, nosebleeds, bruising, and aching joints or bones. Adults suffer gradual or rapid weakness, fever, and night sweats, as well as loss of weight and appetite. Bruising of the legs and arms may be common, the gums may bleed, and women may have heavy periods. The lymph glands become swollen.

How is it diagnosed?
A diagnosis of leukemia and identification of its subtype will be made from a blood test and a bone marrow biopsy.

A blood film and bone marrow smear will usually clearly show the morphology (shape and features) characteristic of the malignant cell type. If leukemia in the cerebrospinal fluid is suspected, a spinal tap will be carried out under local anesthetic, and some fluid will be drawn by syringe from the sheath surrounding the spinal cord. A geneticist will analyze bone marrow to determine whether the leukemia cells have an abnormal chromosome pattern.

What are the treatment options?

It is important to find out which cell type is leukemic and whether there is a particular chromosomal pattern, because both of these factors have an influence on the treatment that will be given. Flow cytometry (p. 107) both confirms leukemia (by measuring different proteins on the surface of cells) and monitors how many leukemic cells are in the blood or bone marrow. A major advance in research has been the recognition of varying responses to treatment and differing treatment requirements according to the genetic abnormalities of the leukemia subtype. Polymerase chain reaction (PCR) technologies are used to do this (p. 109).

ACUTE LYMPHOBLASTIC LEUKEMIA

This is the most common childhood cancer, with the highest incidence at about five years of age. It is rare after age 15. This cancer is characterized by an excess of immature lymphocytes (a type of white cell) in the bone marrow and blood. In most cases, the cell involved has features of a B and T cell precursor (a cell that in normal development could turn into either a B or a T cell), and most of the remaining cases are T cell leukemias.

What are the causes?

Often no cause can be identified; the cancer does not appear to be genetic in origin.

What are the symptoms?

Symptoms include tiredness, weight loss, fever, bleeding gums, and unusual bruising. Bone and joint pain and possibly abdominal pain caused by an enlarged spleen may also be noticeable. Because the normal balance of immune cells is upset in this disease, signs of infection may also be present. If the leukemia has reached the cerebrospinal fluid, headache and nausea may also be symptoms.

How is it diagnosed?

Samples of blood and bone marrow will be taken, from which the hematologist will be able to identify the leukemic cell type, and the geneticist will be able to show whether there is a significant chromosome abnormality present that may influence the treatment.

What are the treatment options?

Treatment with chemotherapy is usually started within a couple of days of diagnosis. Blood and bone marrow samples will be taken regularly to verify that the treatment is appropriate. The cure rate for children is now excellent. If the leukemia does return, chemotherapy is given again, perhaps more intensively, and is sometimes followed by stem cell transplantation.

ACUTE MYELOID LEUKEMIA

This is cancer of an immature bone marrow white cell type. It is less obviously age related than acute lymphoblastic leukemia, and anyone may be afflicted, from the very young to the elderly.

What are the symptoms?

Symptoms are usually tiredness, fever, and weight loss. There may also be bleeding from the gums and bruising anywhere on the body.

How is it diagnosed?

The doctor will take account of the symptoms and arrange for blood and bone marrow tests. These will reveal the type of white cell involved and whether there is a particular chromosome abnormality. From this information, the hematologist or oncologist will make a decision as to the type of treatment to be given. The presence of certain chromosome changes in the leukemic cells indicates a statistically better or worse prognosis.

What are the treatment options?

The initial treatment is chemotherapy, although sometimes this is not enough to control the leukemia. Stem cell transplantation must then be carried out. Acute myeloid leukemia can actually be caused by high-dose chemotherapy or radiation given as treatment for previous cancers such as lymphoma. This potential was recognized relatively recently, and now high-dose regimens are given only when unavoidable.

CHRONIC LYMPHOCYTIC LEUKEMIA

This type of leukemia, which affects the lymphocytes in the blood and in the lymph nodes, is most common among older people.

What are the causes?

The causes of most cases of chronic lymphocytic leukemias (CLL) are unknown. A minority of cases of CLL involving T cells are caused by a virus called HTLV-1, which is relatively common in Japan and the Caribbean. HTLV-1 is a distant cousin of HIV. Both viruses infect T cells, but the big difference is that HIV destroys T cells (eventually causing AIDS) whereas HTLV-1 makes T cells malignant, and they then increase in number.

What are the symptoms?

In many patients, chronic lymphocytic leukemia does not show any symptoms at all; in others, it causes swollen lymph nodes or spleen and fever. Sometimes CLL causes a secondary immune deficiency, with antibody deficiency (leading to chest infections) and impaired T cells (leading to problems such as shingles). CLL can also cause an autoimmune attack of the red cells and platelets; it is one cause of immune thrombocytopenia, ITP (p. 146). Unlike other leukemias, full-blown bone marrow failure is rare in cases of CLL.

How is it diagnosed?

The first step in the diagnosis of chronic lymphocytic leukemia is the discovery of a raised lymphocyte count, as part of the complete blood count. The CLL may turn up as an unexpected diagnosis when the blood count is done for other reasons—for example, before an operation. The lymphocyte count can also be raised in cases of infection, and the hematologist needs to distinguish these from CLL. This distinction is usually made by flow cytometry (p. 107).

Generally, lymphocytes responding to infections are a mixture of B and T cells. In CLL, the situation is quite different. In about 95 percent of cases of CLL, all the cells will be either B cells or T cells. Flow cytometry is so good at diagnosing CLL that bone marrow testing is often not required for this type of leukemia. Flow cytometry can also count the number of malignant cells, so it is possible to assess a patient's response to treatment.

What are the treatment options?

About half of all cases of chronic lymphocytic leukemia are discovered when a blood count is done for another reason; in these cases, patients do not present any symptoms, and often no treatment is required. For patients who do experience symptoms, courses of steroids can be helpful even if the leukemia is not cured.

CHRONIC MYELOID LEUKEMIA

This is cancer of the immature white cells that produce neutrophils. It can affect people of any age.

What are the causes?

Chronic myeloid leukemia (CML) can occur after radiation or after administration of chemotherapy to treat another form of cancer. In most cases of CML, characteristic damaged chromosomes are present. These are referred to as the Philadelphia chromosome, and the genetic mutations that occur as a result are the cause of CML. When CML switches to a more aggressive form, more mutations or chromosomal damage are usually seen.

What are the symptoms?

Symptoms such as an enlarged spleen (splenomegaly, see p. 153) or bone marrow failure (p. 138) are common. The bone marrow failure may be quite mild, with modest

What makes cancer cells so different from other cells?

Malignant cells differ from normal healthy body cells in two crucial characteristics. First, they are monoclonal—that is, all the malignant cells in a single tumor are genetically identical. Genetic changes make the malignant cell inclined to keep dividing and producing many more malignant cells. Second, they are immortal. Most cells have a specific life span: For example, neutrophils survive for only a few days and then built-in mechanisms kill the cells. In malignancy, genetic changes affect the mechanisms that control the life span of the cell. For example, the chromosomal damage (called the Philadelphia chromosome) that causes chronic myeloid leukemia makes the cells immortal, able to continue dividing and multiplying indefinitely.

Several genetic changes, or mutations, are usually required to make cells malignant. Sometimes there is a genetic basis for these changes, which is why some cancers run in families. For example, some individuals inherit an inability to repair defects in DNA. Infections may be involved in making cells malignant: The Epstein-Barr virus is implicated in lymphoma, and the *Helicobacter pylori* bacterium has been linked to stomach cancer, for example.

ASK THE EXPERT

fatigue, for example, being a symptom of anemia. CML has a tendency to transform to a more aggressive disease, similar to acute myeloid leukemia.

How is it diagnosed?
Chronic myeloid leukemia is suggested by finding a very high neutrophil count in a blood sample, and abnormal neutrophils on a blood film. Bone marrow examination may be required. Cytogenetic testing of blood or bone marrow will probably show the Philadelphia chromosome in the majority of cases.

What are the treatment options?
Chemotherapy is used to treat CML. Strong chemotherapy followed by a stem cell transplant is frequently needed, but treatment can only slow the disease, not cure it.

LYMPHOMA
A solid cancer of the lymphocytes, different from leukemia (which can be thought of as liquid cancer in the blood).

Lymphoma generally occurs in the lymph nodes, the home of lymphocytes, but because lymphocytes can move around, it can occur anywhere in the body. There are various types of lymphoma. Hodgkin's disease (p. 145) is one major type; all the others are referred to as non-Hodgkin's lymphoma (NHL) or simply as lymphoma. Burkitt's lymphoma (p. 139) is a special kind of non-Hodgkin's lymphoma.

The incidence of NHL is increasing steadily through its rise in frequency in patients on immunosuppressive drugs or with HIV. The normal immune system can recognize and kill lymphoma cells; when the immune system is damaged by HIV or drugs, lymphoma can occur.

What are the symptoms?
The first indication of NHL is usually a lump or swollen painless lymph gland. This may be accompanied by weight loss, tiredness, and unusual sweating at night.

How is it diagnosed?
If the doctor suspects NHL, the patient is referred to a hospital for a biopsy of the lump or lymph gland. A piece of the lump is taken under general anesthetic, or a needle biopsy is performed. The lump is then tested for signs of abnormal cells. A blood test is also done, and a sample of bone marrow taken to check if the lymphoma is present in the marrow. CT or MRI scans are done to see if the lymphoma has spread to other parts of the body. If NHL is confirmed, the extent of the disease will be determined, and the stage of the disease is designated on a scale of one to four.

What are the treatment options?
Chemotherapy and radiation are generally used to treat lymphoma. A complete cure is possible for some people; in other cases, treatment relieves the symptoms and can prolong life for several years.

MYALGIC ENCEPHALITIS (ME)
See Chronic fatigue syndrome, p. 140.

MYELOMA
A cancer of specialized B lymphocytes known as plasma cells that tends to affect elderly people.

Normally, plasma cells secrete antibodies (also known as immunoglobulins) and play a key role in protecting against infection. In multiple myeloma, monoclonal plasma cells secrete only one kind of antibody and grow uncontrollably, taking over the bone marrow.

What are the causes?
The cause is uncertain, although because myeloma tends to run in families there may be a genetic element to it.

What are the symptoms?
Myeloma starts in the bone marrow and as it spreads, causes widespread bone damage, bone pain, and fractures. Useful antibody production is impaired, and sufferers are prone to infections such as chest infection.

How is it diagnosed?
When myeloma is suspected, electrophoresis (the study of the movement of charged particles such as proteins) is carried out to see if there is abnormal immunoglobulin in the blood or urine. A bone marrow examination is required to confirm the diagnosis.

What are the treatment options?
Some myelomas grow very slowly and require no treatment. Other, more serious cases require chemotherapy; this may suppress the myeloma for several years or sometimes even cure it.

NON-HODGKIN'S LYMPHOMA
See *Lymphoma, p. 150.*

PERNICIOUS ANEMIA
An autoimmune disease that results in a deficiency of vitamin B_{12} and anemia.

What is the cause?
Vitamin B_{12} is present in a wide range of foods, so it is unusual for deficiency to result from a lack of vitamin B_{12} in the diet. However, vitamin B_{12} is not easily absorbed from the digestive tract. Stomach cells called gastric parietal cells help absorb the vitamin by secreting a protein known as intrinsic factor. In pernicious anemia, the immune system makes antibodies that kill off both gastric parietal cells and intrinsic factor, blocking normal absorption of the vitamin.

What are the symptoms?
Patients with pernicious anemia are usually anemic (p. 134). Sometimes, because B_{12} is required by the nervous system, they may feel tingling or loss of balance.

How is it diagnosed?
A complete blood count will show that the red cells are abnormally large. The diagnosis is confirmed by low levels of vitamin B_{12} in the blood as well as antibodies against gastric parietal cells and intrinsic factor.

What are the treatment options?
Vitamin B_{12} injections, given every month or so throughout the patient's life, ensure a good outlook.

RAYNAUD'S PHENOMENON
A painful condition that can occur when the hands or feet become very cold.

What are the causes?
This condition is caused by poor blood supply to fingers and toes. In cold temperatures, arteries constrict, making the problem worse. Rarely, the condition can be caused by an underlying disease such as myeloma (p. 150), in which blood can be so thick and sticky that it can't flow into the fingers, or SLE (p. 154), in which blood can't flow normally through inflamed arteries. The condition is a common side effect of beta blocker drugs used for high blood pressure. Women are particularly susceptible to mild Raynaud's phenomenon.

What are the symptoms?
The hands and toes turn very pale and become painful when cold; in severe cases, the fingers or toes may turn blue. When the patient warms up again, the fingers and toes turn red and may throb or tingle. In extreme cases, the blood supply becomes so damaged that the tissue in the fingers and toes may die and become gangrenous. In most cases of Raynaud's phenomenon, however, although the condition can be distressing, it does not cause gangrene.

How is it diagnosed?
A blood test will be taken to rule out any underlying disease. A normal protein electrophoresis (p. 110) will be used to check for myeloma, and a normal autoantibody test will eliminate the possibility of SLE.

What are the treatment options?
Medications that dilate blood vessels, such as calcium channel blockers, are often effective in treating the condition. But prevention is the best option: Patients should avoid exposing the fingers, toes, and face to the cold. Wearing gloves, warm socks, and boots outdoors should help. Oven mitts can be used when taking food from the fridge or freezer. Sufferers should get help to stop smoking because smoking also causes arterial disease. In extreme progressive cases, an operation to cut the sympathetic nerves may be performed, but this provides relief for only a year or two.

SEVERE COMBINED IMMUNODEFICIENCY (SCID)
This is not a single deficiency but a group of inherited immunodeficiencies affecting babies.

What are the causes?
There are about ten different known genetic causes of SCID. Some are X-chromosome-linked, which means that the defective gene can be passed from the mother; others are autosomal recessive—that is, both parents must carry the gene to pass the condition to their offspring. The mutations that cause SCID all affect proteins that are normally found in T cells.

What are the symptoms?
Babies with SCID become ill very soon after birth. They have no T cells and so are vulnerable to the same range of infections as patients with AIDS. They develop infections

and rashes and fail to put on weight. These symptoms can be very vague and so are not always recognized quickly by doctors.

How is it diagnosed?
SCID can be rapidly diagnosed by doing a complete blood count, which will show that the number of lymphocytes is very low. Then a T cell count will be done; it usually shows that there are no T cells in the blood.

What are the treatment options?
Babies with SCID need to be protected from infections. In the past, they were kept in large plastic "bubbles" to protect them—the celebrated "boy in the bubble" was a child with SCID. These days, with a better understanding of the problem, antibiotics can be given to prevent infections for several months at a time, and bubbles are no longer required. Nonetheless, babies with SCID need to be given a new immune system if they are to survive. This can be done by stem cell transplant, but only if there is a suitable donor. An alternative is gene therapy, which has been successfully used for one form of SCID—gamma chain deficiency.

SEPTICEMIA
Previously known as blood poisoning, septicemia is a condition in which bacteria grow in the blood.

What are the causes?
Bacteria should never be present in the blood; if they are, the body's defenses must have been damaged. Septicemia commonly occurs when skin is damaged by severe burns, reflecting the skin's role as the biggest barrier to infection.

Septicemia also happens if parts of the immune system are impaired. The cells responsible for clearing bacteria from blood are called phagocytes. These cells literally eat up bacteria and then kill them; they include neutrophils that circulate in the blood and other cells in the spleen.

Phagocytes can be damaged in different ways—many of them medically induced. For example, if the neutrophil count is very low (neutropenia), often as a result of chemotherapy for cancer, septicemia can complicate what normally would be trivial skin infections. Such patients are usually given advice on avoiding infections and told to seek help quickly if they develop early symptoms of septicemia. If the spleen is removed, there is also a very high risk of septicemia; indeed, the risk is so great that patients are often advised to stay on antibiotics for life.

What are the symptoms?
The symptoms of septicemia include fevers, sweating and shivering. Septicemia damages the body's mechanism for maintaining blood pressure, and as blood pressure falls, the patient may lose consciousness and the kidneys may fail.

How is it diagnosed?
Blood cultures to confirm that bacteria are actually growing in the blood can be done, but septicemia needs to be diagnosed quickly.

What are the treatment options?
As soon as septicemia is suspected, intravenous antibiotics are given to control the infection. Special measures, including intravenous fluids and drugs, are used to try to improve blood pressure. If the infection is rapidly controlled, patients will make a complete recovery.

SHINGLES
A local skin infection caused by the herpes virus varicella zoster.

Single (never repeated) outbreaks of mild shingles can happen when the immune system is temporarily suppressed by stress or old age. More severe or repeated attacks of shingles can be a sign of more serious immune deficiency, caused by HIV infection (p. 144) or chronic lymphocytic leukemia, for example (p. 148).

What are the causes?
Shingles is caused by the varicella zoster virus (VZV) which causes chicken pox when it first infects people, usually in childhood. The T cells of the immune system bring the chicken pox under control after a few days, but the virus remains hidden in the nervous system.

What are the symptoms?
If the immune system is damaged, the virus breaks out again, causing a painful rash in a beltlike pattern around one side of the trunk. Sometimes shingles also affects one side of the face, and it can damage vision.

How is it diagnosed?
Shingles may be suspected from the patient's history and the type and position of the rash. A definitive diagnosis can be reached by culturing samples of spots in a laboratory.

What are the treatment options?

Treatment with the antiviral drug aciclovir can reduce the length of a shingles attack. Painkillers are usually needed because the pain can be severe and it can persist after the rash has disappeared. Occasionally, there may be permanent numbness or tingling of the skin at the site of the attack.

SICKLE CELL DISEASE

An inherited form of anemia in which a large number of red blood cells become sickle shaped.

Sickle cell anemia is most common in those of sub-Saharan African and Mediterranean descent.

What are the causes?

The disease is caused by a mutation in the hemoglobin gene. When the amount of oxygen in the blood is low, abnormal hemoglobin molecules form crystals that damage red cells, resulting in anemia. Damaged red cells also block blood vessels, causing oxygen levels in the blood to fall even further.

The severity of the sickle syndrome depends on the number of abnormal genes. A patient with one abnormal gene (for instance, someone who has inherited a normal gene from the mother and an abnormal gene from the father) has a less severe disease called sickle cell trait. There are symptoms only when oxygen levels are low, such as when flying in unpressurized airplanes. People with the more severe sickle cell disease have inherited two sets of abnormal hemoglobin genes and can develop symptoms at any time. It may be that sickle cell trait is an advantage in Africa; the malaria parasite finds it much harder to infect red cells that contain this hemoglobin, so carrying one set of abnormal genes may give some protection from malaria.

What are the symptoms?

Anemia and bone pain caused by damaged red blood cells blocking the blood vessels.

How is it diagnosed?

The abnormal hemoglobin can be detected by carrying out hemoglobin electrophoresis.

What are the treatment options?

Antibiotics are given to prevent infections. Blood transfusions may be an option, and research is ongoing into stem cell and bone marrow transplant for sufferers.

ON THE CUTTING EDGE

Using umbilical cord blood to treat sickle cell disease

A baby's umbilical cord is rich in stem cells, the building blocks of the immune system and whole blood. In 1998, researchers in Atlanta took blood from the cord of an unrelated baby and gave it to a 12-year-old boy with sickle cell disease. The boy had experienced his first stroke at five years old, and despite regular blood transfusions was in constant pain and at risk of a second stroke. Normal red cells were produced by stem cells in the cord blood, and the boy's symptoms improved. Unlike bone marrow transplant, cord blood doesn't have to be a good match to be effective; because the cells in cord blood are immature, a host does not recognize them as foreign and reject them. The belief was that the cord blood would enable the patient to manufacture healthy blood cells.

SPLENOMEGALY

This term simply means "big spleen" and describes the swelling of the spleen caused by a range of illnesses.

The spleen is an organ about the size of a fist in the upper abdomen. One of its roles is to act as a filter: It can remove bacteria from the blood, for example. It also removes old red cells, neutrophils, and platelets. If the spleen is enlarged, it may start removing healthy cells from the blood, causing red cell, platelet, and neutrophil counts to fall. An enlarged spleen is also at higher risk of rupture after injury.

What are the causes?

The spleen becomes enlarged transiently in some cases of infectious mononucleosis, but can become more permanently enlarged in lymphoma and leukemia, when it fills up with abnormal blood cells. In some forms of liver disease, the spleen swells because the liver increases the amount of blood flowing through it. There are several other forms of splenomegaly, including immune thrombocytopenia, ITP (p. 146).

What are the symptoms?

The prime symptom is the enlarged spleen, but general symptoms of infection such as fever may also be present.

How is it diagnosed?
Physical examination and medical history of the patient will point to a diagnosis.

What are the treatment options?
If the cause of splenomegaly cannot be treated, the spleen may need to be surgically removed.

SYSTEMIC LUPUS ERYTHEMATOSUS
An autoimmune disease in which the immune system makes antibodies against DNA.

What are the causes?
DNA can leak from damaged cells and enter the blood, where antibodies bind on it. A DNA antibody circulating in the blood triggers damage. In systemic lupus erythematosus (SLE), the damage takes the form of inflamed blood vessels, particularly at key sites such as the skin, joints, and kidneys. Because SLE causes blood vessel inflammation, it is classed as a type of vasculitis.

SLE tends to run in families. In most cases, the genetic basis for this inheritance is not known, but in some cases, patients inherit a deficiency in the complement proteins. Like most autoimmune diseases, although there is a strong genetic risk of getting the disease, an environmental trigger is also required. In some women at least, this trigger may be taking the contraceptive pill or another medication.

What are the symptoms?
SLE tends to affect young women. Initial symptoms may include rashes on parts of the skin exposed to the sun, Raynaud's phenomenon, and joint pain. Like many autoimmune diseases, SLE can stay relatively mild or become more severe, in which case there can be kidney and brain damage, blood clots, and miscarriages.

How is it diagnosed?
Lupus is hard to diagnose and easy to miss. Doctors need to know about all of the symptoms. A special autoantibody test (the antinuclear antibody test—98 percent of SLE sufferers have this antibody in their blood) is used to pinpoint a diagnosis of SLE.

What are the treatment options?
The treatment of SLE depends on the severity of each individual case. For mild cases, antiinflammatory drugs may be enough; in more severe cases, immunosuppressive drugs may have to be given. Although most symptoms can be controlled, SLE does not go away and most patients require treatment for life.

THALASSEMIA
An inherited condition in which mutations in the hemoglobin gene make it impossible for the body to make hemoglobin.

Thalassemia is common in people from the Mediterranean region, Asia, and some parts of Africa. It may be that, as with sickle cell trait (p. 153), having one abnormal gene offers some protection from malaria.

About 100,000 babies worldwide are born with severe forms of thalassemia each year.

What are the causes?
The mild form of thalassemia is caused by inheriting just one abnormal gene. In this case, it is still possible for the patient to make red blood cells. People who inherit two abnormal genes have severe problems making red cells.

What are the symptoms?
People with mild forms of the disease tend to be anemic; for people who inherit two abnormal genes, the anemia is severe. Iron is usually incorporated with hemoglobin, but patients with severe thalassemia cannot make hemoglobin, so iron builds up in the body, poisoning the liver. Blood tests show the presence of the condition.

What are the treatment options?
Regular blood transfusions may be necessary for more severe cases, with antibiotics to treat infection. Repeated transfusions, however, can lead to iron overload, so drugs are needed to correct this. Bone marrow transplant offers a cure, but there are few suitable donors. It is hoped that gene therapy may offer the possibility of a cure.

VASCULITIS
This term applies to a group of diseases that are caused by inflammation of the blood vessels.

What are the causes?
There are many different types of vasculitis, which are generally caused by the immune system. Each one tends to affect certain groups and produces distinct symptoms.

Sometimes inflammation of blood vessels is caused by mixtures of antibody and target molecules circulating in the blood. SLE (p. 154) is an example of damage by what is referred to as immune complexes. Immune complexes can occur after sore throats caused by bacteria, when complexes of antibody and bacterial protein circulate in the blood.

In other instances, the immune system makes a direct attack on the blood vessels as a type of autoimmunity.

Little is known about the causes of temporal arteritis, a common vasculitis affecting elderly people, which results in inflammation in the blood vessels in the head. Behçet's disease is another vasculitis, which affects people along the old Silk Road that extended from the Middle East to China. For both temporal arteritis and Behçet's syndrome, there must be a specific cause to affect such particular groups. As with all autoimmune problems, it is likely that there is a genetic basis for these diseases but that an environmental trigger (maybe an infection) is needed to initiate them.

What are the symptoms?
In cases of immune complexes circulating in the bloodstream, damage to the kidneys is likely. Severe headaches are the usual symptom of temporal arteritis, but blindness or stroke can sometimes develop. In Behçet's syndrome, ulcers form in the mouth and on the genitals, and eye disease and skin and joint problems are characteristic.

How is it diagnosed?
Vasculitis can sometimes be diagnosed on the basis of specific blood tests, for example the antinuclear antibody test in SLE. For other diseases, including Behçet's syndrome and temporal arteritis, there is no specific blood test, and the diagnosis is apparent from the unusual symptoms.

What are the treatment options?
Most types of vasculitis, except those caused by infection, respond well to immunosuppressive drugs. In these cases the outlook is good.

X-LINKED DISORDERS
Genetic disorders resulting from mutations on the X chromosome.

The genetic code is contained in the 23 chromosomes present in most body cells. Each of these chromosomes is present as a pair: one inherited from the mother, the other from the father. For chromosomes 1–22, each member of

the pair looks very similar, although the detailed genetic codes are different. The 23rd chromosome determines the sex of an individual, and the two members of the pair look very different. Chromosome 23 can be an X chromosome or a much smaller Y chromosome. Women have two X chromosomes; men have an X chromosome and a Y chromosome.

When eggs are made in a woman's ovaries, each egg receives just one chromosome from each pair. Because women have two X chromosomes, each egg will receive one of these. Sperm cells produced by men also receive one of each pair of chromosomes. Because men's cells have an X and a Y chromosome, each sperm can be either X or Y. An egg fertilized by an X sperm will make a female (XX) baby; an egg fertilized by a Y sperm will make a male (XY) baby. Because there is a 50 percent chance of either of these happening, about 50 percent of babies are boys and 50 percent are girls.

What are the causes?
Some diseases are the result of mutations on the X chromosome. Women are not usually affected by these diseases because they have two X chromosomes; even if they inherit a mutated X chromosome, this will be balanced by a normal one. Only women can carry X-linked disorders. Men have just one X chromosome, so if they inherit a mutation, it will cause disease.

What are the symptoms?
The symptoms will be particular to the disease. X-linked disorders include chronic granulomatous disease (p. 140), some forms of SCID (p. 151), and antibody deficiency (p. 137). The best-known disease is hemophilia (p. 144), of which a famous example is the family of Queen Victoria, which shows a typical X-linked disease pattern. Victoria was a carrier of hemophilia, as were two daughters and four granddaughters. She also had one affected son, three affected grandsons, and five affected great-grandsons.

How is it diagnosed?
It is now possible for genetic testing to identify a female carrier of these diseases. It is then possible to see if a male fetus is affected, if the carrier wishes.

What are the treatment options?
Treatment for these X-linked conditions aims to relieve the symptoms. A patient's outlook will depend on the particular disease or disorder.

Index

Acknowledgments

Carroll & Brown Limited would also like to thank:

Picture researcher
Sandra Schneider

Production manager
Karol Davies

Production controller
Nigel Reed

Computer management
Paul Stradling

Indexer
Jill Dormon

3-D anatomy
Mirashade/Matt Gould

Illustrators
Andy Baker, Rajeev Doshi/Regraphica, Kevin Jones Associates, Mikki Rain, John Woodcock

Layout and illustration assistance
Joanna Cameron

Photographer
Jules Selmes

Photographic sources
SPL = Science Photo Library

1 SPL
6 *(right)* Getty Images
7 Michael Abbey/SPL
8 *(top left)* CNRI/SPL
8 *(background)* Andrew Syred/SPL
8/9 Getty Images
10 *(top)* Edelmann/SPL
10/11 *(background)* Andrew Syred/SPL
10/11 Dan McCoy/Rainbow/medipics
11 *(left)* Getty Images
11 *(right)* Roy Morsch/Corbis
12 *(background)* Andrew Syred/SPL
12 *(left)* LWA-Stephen Welstead/Corbis
12 *(right)* Tom & Dee McCarthy/ Corbis
13 *(top)* Hank Morgan/SPL
13 CNRI/SPL
14 *(center)* Getty Images
(right) NIBSC/SPL
19 BSIP Meullemiestre/SPL

27 NIBSC/SPL
30 SPL
38 Getty Images
39 *(top, center)* Getty Images
(bottom) Jose Luis Pelaez Inc./ Corbis
40 *(center)* Getty Images
41 Getty Images
42 *(top right)* Getty Images
(4th from top) Getty Images
43 Getty Images
45 *(left)* Getty Images
47 Getty Images
51 John Henley/Corbis
54 *(left, center, bottom)* Getty Images
55 TEK Image/SPL
58 Getty Images
59 *(top, 3rd from top)* Getty Images
62 Tiziana & Gianni Baldizzone/ Corbis
63 *(top)* Getty Images
66 *(bottom)* Getty Images
70 www.tefal.co.uk
75 *(right, 2nd, 3rd from top, bottom)* Getty Images
78 Getty Images
83 Getty Images
84 Getty Images
87 *(left)* Getty Images
87 *(top right)* Sinclair Stammers/SPL
88 Getty Images
90 Sinclair Stammers/SPL
91 London School of Hygiene and Tropical Medicine/SPL
92 Medipics
93 Getty Images
96 *(left)* Dr. Gopal Murti/SPL
(center) TEK Image/SPL
(right) Wellcome Trust Medical Photographic Library
97 Nina Lampen/SPL
100 Dr. Gopal Murti/SPL
103 Wellcome Trust Medical Photographic Library
104 *(top)* Charles Gupton/Corbis
(bottom) Saturn Stills/SPL
105 John Greim/SPL
106 John Radcliffe Hospital/SPL
107 *(top)* Michael Abbey/SPL
(bottom) Geoff Tompkinson/SPL
108 Simon Fraser/Department of Haematology/RVI, Newcastle/SPL
110 TEK Image/SPL
111 Philippe Plailly/Eurelios/SPL
114 *(top)* Cordelia Molloy/SPL
(bottom) Getty Images-Foodpix
115 Jerry Mason/SPL

116 TEK Image/SPL
117 St. Bartholomew's Hospital/SPL
118 Nina Lampen/SPL
119 John Greim/SPL
120 Colin Cuthbert/SPL
121 Colin Cuthbert/SPL
123 Great Ormond Street
124 *(top)* Geoff Tompkinson/SPL
(center) SPL
(bottom) Andrew Syred/SPL
125 *(top)* Andrew Tsiaras/SPL
(bottom) Great Ormond Street
127 Bill Varie/Corbis
129 Copyright 2002, The Regents of the University of Michigan
130 Getty Images
131 Getty Images

Back cover *(center)* Getty Images
(right) TEK Image/SPL

Contact details
Centers for Disease Control
www.cdc.gov

National Institute for Health
www.nih.gov

Organ donation
www.organdonor.gov
www.optn.org
www.shareyourlife.org

Transplant Games
www.transweb.org

American Red Cross
www.redcross.org
1-800-435-7669

619–008–1